Managing Risk in Healthcare Law and Practice

Ge~~~~l Editor

Dr Van

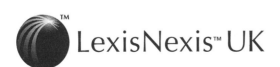

' or befo   ...date shown '

LexisNexis™ UK

Members of the LexisNexis Group worldwide

United Kingdom	LexisNexis UK, a Division of Reed Elsevier (UK) Ltd, 2 Addiscombe Road, CROYDON CR9 5AF
Argentina	LexisNexis Argentina, BUENOS AIRES
Australia	LexisNexis Butterworths, CHATSWOOD, New South Wales
Austria	LexisNexis Verlag ARD Orac GmbH & Co KG, VIENNA
Canada	LexisNexis Butterworths, MARKHAM, Ontario
Chile	LexisNexis Chile Ltda, SANTIAGO DE CHILE
Czech Republic	Nakladatelství Orac sro, PRAGUE
France	Editions du Juris-Classeur SA, PARIS
Germany	LexisNexis Deutschland GmbH, FRANKFURT, MUNSTER
Hong Kong	LexisNexis Butterworths, HONG KONG
Hungary	HVG-Orac, BUDAPEST
India	LexisNexis Butterworths, NEW DELHI
Ireland	LexisNexis, DUBLIN
Italy	Giuffrè Editore, MILAN
Malaysia	Malayan Law Journal Sdn Bhd, KUALA LUMPUR
New Zealand	LexisNexis Butterworths, WELLINGTON
Poland	Wydawnictwo Prawnicze LexisNexis, WARSAW
Singapore	LexisNexis Butterworths, SINGAPORE
South Africa	LexisNexis Butterworths, DURBAN
Switzerland	Stämpfli Verlag AG, BERNE
USA	LexisNexis, DAYTON, Ohio

© Reed Elsevier (UK) Ltd 2004

Published by LexisNexis UK

A CIP Catalogue record for this book is available from the British Library.

ISBN 0 4069 7358 X

Typeset by Columns Design Ltd, Reading, England
Printed and bound in Great Britian by Hobbs the Printers Ltd, Totton, Hampshire

Visit LexisNexis UK at www.lexisnexis.co.uk

Foreword

I have a vision for safer health services, for both patients and staff where all those who have an influence in delivering care have safety at the front of their minds, where care becomes systematically better and safer for patients and where decisions increasingly take into account the wider implications for safety.

And I'm very pleased to see that this vision is gaining worldwide momentum.

But this has not always been the case. Until comparatively recently in the history of our own National Health Service (NHS), the quality and safety of services were not a widely debated subject outside those with an academic or specialist interest. Quality was, historically, an implicit rather than an explicit part of day-to-day service delivery. Management attention was focused on achieving higher activity levels and using resources more efficiently.

Since the late 1990s, a systematic drive to improve the quality of NHS care, has been based, at its core, upon the concepts of risk management and clinical governance. This has established a fundamental principle that all NHS organisations should have in place proper systems to assure and improve the quality of services they provide for the benefit of both staff and patients. Clinical governance is underpinned by a statutory duty of quality enshrined in an Act of Parliament; there are long established statutory requirements for the safety of staff and the environment in which care is delivered.

A key strand of the forthcoming national standards defines the quality of care we can expect from the NHS. Good quality goes hand in hand with good risk management from which patients, staff and healthcare organisations can benefit.

This emphasis on safety requires a big shift for a hospital or a primary care service. It requires transformation in culture, operating systems and working practices. A full appreciation of the vulnerability of the systems of an organisation, and a refocusing of all activity to the needs and experience of the patient are also needed, coupled with an approach based upon learning from error not blame and punishment.

Patient safety and risk management are no longer the domain of specialist 'risk managers'. Safety is everybody's business.

Consequently, I welcome the second edition of this book. It provides an excellent review of this important field, offering readers new to the subject as well as existing managers and specialists a clear and comprehensive guide to the assessment and management of risk in health care.

Sir Liam Donaldson
Chief Medical Officer, Department of Health, April 2004

About the Authors

Dr Vanessa L Mayatt, BSc PhD DipOHS FRSH MIOSH RSP

Vanessa is an independent risk management consultant and member of the Boards of the Public Health Laboratory Service and the newly created Health Protection Agency. She is a member of the visitor panel of the Joint Committee on Postgraduate Training for General Practice. Previous posts held include health and safety director for PPP Healthcare and AXA Assistance, healthcare practice leader for Marsh, health and safety practice leader for Marsh, research fellow and visiting fellow at Salford University's European Occupational Health and Safety Law Research Centre and NHS trust unit director for Sedgwick. Prior to joining Sedgwick, she was HM principal specialist inspector of health and safety within HSE. Vanessa has worked with the healthcare sector in her various roles since 1984 and has extensive experience of helping the sector to manage risk. She has lectured widely on risk management and corporate governance including the management of occupational health and safety and clinical risk. She has many publications to her name. Vanessa has been a member of the *Health Care Risk Report* editorial board since 1995.

Mary Burrows, MBE BSc MBA LLM

Mary is chief executive of Northampton Primary Care Trust, which commissions and provides services for the local population. She is an American citizen but has spent the last twelve years in the UK. During this time she has worked mainly in acute hospital care, spending nine years at the Oxford Radcliffe Hospitals NHS Trust in senior management positions before moving into primary care in 2000. Mary has over 20 years experience of clinical practice and management in the UK and US. She has been a member of the Health and Safety Commission's Health Services Advisory Committee and, in 1996, was awarded a MBE in recognition of her risk management achievements in the NHS.

Janet Martin, BA Chartered FCIPD

Janet is Associate Director, Employment with SCOPE, a not for profit NHS trading agency providing specialist advice and guidance to NHS and independent healthcare employers on employment and human resource issues. She also works within the Eastern Deanery as a human resource consultant which involves her in the national medical workforce agenda, the appointment of doctors in training, assessment and appeal arrangements and the provision of training in equality and interview skills. Janet has worked in the NHS in a number of human resource roles dealing with employment relations and organisational change issues. She is a member of the NHSP *Employment Law Register* editorial board, and a nominated member of the NHS national group providing public sector input to *CEEP UK*, a European Social Partner organisation.

Graham E Offord, MCBIS MBCI AIRM

Graham has worked in the risk management arena for 15 years. He is Managing Consultant of Offrisk Consulting Ltd. Over the years he has been instrumental in the implementation of business continuity plans across various sectors throughout the UK and Europe. Graham's particular areas of expertise include Board Room strategic risk, business continuity policy, risk and impact analysis, recovery strategy, plan development and implementation, training and plan rehearsal, all as part of a comprehensive development of an organisation's awareness of risk management by its people.

Trevor Payne, MSc FBIFM

Trevor is Director of estates and facilities at the Great Western Hospital (Swindon and Marlborough NHS Trust), a first wave PFI hospital – one of the newest flagship NHS hospitals. He is setting up an informed client function to effectively manage the PFI contract. He has a professional engineering background having trained in both Electrical and Plant Engineering and subsequently gaining a MSc in Facilities Management at Strathclyde Graduate Business School. Trevor is a seasoned lecturer and presenter of papers in international fora. He has also written and contributed to a number of books in his field. He is a member of the editorial board of *Facilities Management*. Trevor is a fellow of the BIFM and Chair of the BIFM Healthcare sector forum, he was awarded the title facilities manager of the year for 2002/3.

John Tingle, BA Law Hons Cert Ed (Dist) MEd Barrister

John is a Reader in Health Law, Nottingham Law School, and Director of the Centre for Health Law, The Nottingham Trent University. His current research interests include the legal aspects of risk management and clinical governance. He has also widely researched the area of the expanded role of the nurse. He was editor of the monthly journal *Health Care Risk Report* for seven years until May 2001. His current publications include:

- *Law and Nursing*, 2nd Edition with Jean McHale, 2001, Butterworth Heinemann, Oxford.

- *Healthcare Law: The Impact of the Human Rights Act 1998*, Co-Editor with Austen Garwood-Gowers and Tom Lewis, 2001, Cavendish Publishing, London.

- *Clinical Guidelines: Law, Policy and Practice*, Co-Editor with Charles Foster, 2002, Cavendish Publishing, London.

- *Nursing Law and Ethics*, 2nd Edition with Alan Cribb, 2002, Blackwell Publishing, Oxford.

John is also responsible for teaching the clinical negligence and clinical risk management components in the Nottingham Law School's LLM Health Law Programme launched in 2001.

Contents

Contents

Chapter 1
General Introduction

Introduction   1.1

Risk management is central to the effective running of any organisation. Within the healthcare sector, risk management is ever more topical. The continued incidents associated with healthcare delivery, where risk has been poorly managed and patients harmed, are almost too many to mention. The intense media coverage of these incidents repeatedly draws public attention to failures in healthcare delivery, whether isolated incidents involving one patient, or poor practice over time involving many patients. Whilst newspapers are sold on the strength of these stories, no one else wins, especially not patients, healthcare organisations or the individuals working within them. This alone should be a strong motivator for effective risk management.

Why is managing risk important?   1.2

Organisations operate against the backdrop of many externally driven requirements to manage risk. These include corporate governance, insurance-related risk management programmes and legal duties. For healthcare organisations, controls assurance, clinical governance, the NHS LA, CNST, NICE, CHAI, HPRA, NPSA and HSE initiatives all need to be added. These many external pressures require the implementation of best practice in managing healthcare organisations and their attendant risks.

External pressures apart, there are other good reasons for managing risk and there are dividends to be reaped from doing so. Increasingly, healthcare organisations are seeing the benefit of managing risk in the quality of patient care, in staff/patient relationships, in staff morale and also financially. Whilst the nature of the external pressures ensures that managing risk is not optional, a genuine organisation-wide belief that risk management is central to looking after patients, staff and ensuring business survival is the best motivator.

Keeping abreast of changes   1.3

Managing risk in healthcare is a fast-moving field. The precise nature and specific requirements of the various external drivers are subject to continual change and development. The pace of these changes is swift. Risk management is an iterative

1

process necessitating constant endeavour to secure ever better standards. Staff working in healthcare organisations as risk management professionals or with responsibility for managing risk, therefore, have a sizeable task to keep abreast of developments on all fronts, to understand what has to be done and then to secure effective implementation.

Aims of this book   1.4

The first edition of this publication originated from a desire to provide a comprehensive and up-to-date steer through the key legal and best practice requirements relevant to managing risk in the healthcare sector. In the two years since the first edition was published many developments have taken place. In line with these developments each of the chapters in the first edition have been updated for this new edition. The overall aim of the handbook is therefore to continue to provide up-to-date guidance on managing specific areas of risk.

The handbook has been written from a practical standpoint by individuals who are both expert in managing risk and have extensive experience of the successful implementation of risk management initiatives in healthcare organisations. All the contributors have set out to demystify the complexities and challenges that are encountered when embarking upon or further developing risk management initiatives. There is much reinvention of the wheel in devising risk management initiatives in the healthcare sector. This handbook aspires to set out the expert views of the various contributors so that experience is shared and healthcare organisations can more efficiently enhance the means by which they manage risk in practice.

Structure of the book

Key references and guidance   1.5

Current key documents and guidance, such as Department of Health reports, as well as essential references are set out in **APPENDIX 1**. At the end of each chapter, other main reference sources are listed. A glossary of the main terms used throughout the chapters is in **APPENDIX 2**.

Managing risk   1.6

The guidance commences at **CHAPTER 2**. This chapter, written by Mary Burrows, contains general guidance on managing risk. For those new to this field, this is an important chapter to start with; it sets the scene for the subsequent chapters. For those more experienced in risk management, this chapter should still prove interesting and useful, as it contains many practical pointers to achieving best practice. The chapter explains the relationship between risk management and the related initiatives of governance, controls assurance and quality. This is done in order to encourage a combined approach to these various initiatives rather than dealing with each separately.

Managing organisational change   1.7

CHAPTER 3 is a new chapter for the second edition, written by Janet Martin and contains material on the Private Finance Initiative (PFI) from myself. The healthcare sector and the NHS in particular is subject to perpetual organisational change. Change, irrespective of scale, can lead to risk. Developments such as PFI, *Agenda for Change*, and the creation of different types of NHS trusts are all associated with risk. This chapter deals with most of the major change programmes currently impinging upon the healthcare sector and the diverse ways that risk may, in consequence, arise.

Incident reporting   1.8

One of the most important aspects of managing risk is the recording of incidents, their analysis to check performance and identify priorities and then investigation to learn lessons and implement change. In recognition of the importance of this aspect of managing risk, this topic is addressed next in **CHAPTER 4**. In this chapter, Mary Burrows covers an area with which many complex and multi-sited organisations struggle both within and outside the healthcare sector, and, consequently, waste much time and energy on. The chapter straddles all areas of risk and will therefore have wide appeal to individuals with risk management responsibilities as well as those with a general interest. The chapter is practically based and contains many excellent tips for the successful implementation of incident recording systems. It also addresses the National Patient Safety Agency (NPSA) requirements for reporting.

The so-called blame culture, whilst not unique to healthcare, has undoubtedly played its part in reducing levels of reported incidents, the factual accuracy of reports and the ability to learn lessons. **CHAPTER 4** explains the importance of establishing a blame-free culture and how this can be achieved in practice.

Clinical risk management   1.9

John Tingle, who has published widely on clinical risk management, is a new contributor to the second edition. **CHAPTER 5** deals specifically with the management of clinical risk, although the emphasis is different from the first edition. The chapter concentrates on clinical negligence and governance and the role of key organisations in this area of risk including the NPSA.

Incidents of clinical negligence continue to attract significant media attention and are often associated with claims for compensation. The number of claims has steadily increased over the last decade as indeed have the value of settlements, particularly, but not exclusively, in obstetric cases. Failing to manage clinical risk does therefore cost the healthcare sector dearly, both in financial terms and in terms of the impact on individuals – both patients and their families, and clinicians, their families and colleagues.

NHS trusts in England have been members of the Clinical Negligence Scheme for Trusts (CNST) since its inception in the early 1990s. This is a major initiative in the clinical risk management arena. Awareness of the CNST's risk management standards both for CNST members and organisations outside of England is clearly important in developing approaches to managing clinical risk. **CHAPTER 5** therefore provides some background in relation to the CNST and the latest developments with its risk management standards.

Managing health, safety and environmental risks   1.10

In **CHAPTER 6**, I deal with the management of health, safety and environmental risks. This updated chapter covers the diverse nature of these risks in healthcare organisations and the consequences of failing to manage them effectively. The principles of effective management and how to establish management systems are also explored. Legislation and good practice guidance in this field is under constant development. The requirements of the main pieces of current legislation are addressed, together with how to comply with these legal requirements. There are several major initiatives in the health, safety and environmental arena that are currently vital to incorporate into any strategy to tackle these areas of risk. These major initiatives are covered together with the anticipated changes in corporate manslaughter legislation.

New material has been incorporated into this chapter on some of the HSE prosecutions that have been taken in the healthcare sector. This has been done to facilitate sharing of the lessons to be learnt from the circumstances. Some of the topical and significant areas of risk for healthcare staff are also covered. In many healthcare organisations, health, safety and environmental risks are separated from measures to address other areas of risk, in particular clinical risk. Arguments are put forward for merging approaches to these two areas and some of the consequences of failing to do so are highlighted.

Managing the physical environment   1.11

The challenges to managing the physical environment and the detail of good management in this area are the focus of Trevor Payne in **CHAPTER 7**. Healthcare is delivered from a diverse range of settings in terms of size, complexity, age, design and maintenance standards. The nature and quality of the healthcare environment can have a direct bearing on the wellbeing of staff and patients. Indeed, if the physical environment is not up to standard, lives can be placed at risk, as has happened in the past. Estates and facilities management is a specialised field, subject to rapid change and is therefore no different from other areas of risk associated with healthcare delivery. Outsourcing, insourcing, PFI-funded developments and Public/Private Partnerships (PPP) are all part of the current territory of specialists in this field. Managing contractors and consortium relationships are challenges for any organisation, but are nonetheless crucial to get right so that money is not wasted, project deadlines are achieved and high quality patient care delivery is assured. This chapter includes new material on the PFI and the implications for estates and facilities management.

Service continuity management 1.12

Over recent years, the healthcare sector has experienced a number of major incidents. These have included multiple deaths from an outbreak of Legionnaires' disease, hospital-acquired infection affecting both patients and staff, and collapse of patient administration systems. Whilst these major incidents are not daily occurrences, they do unfortunately reoccur and on each occasion have a major impact upon service delivery. In **CHAPTER 8**, Graham Offord tackles service continuity planning, the impact of disasters within healthcare and resourcing for disaster recovery. Successful service continuity management requires input from individuals with differing backgrounds and skills. This chapter contains good practice advice that will appeal to a diverse range of roles in the healthcare sector.

Managing people 1.13

The final chapter deals with managing people. People are any organisation's most important asset and this is never more true than within the NHS – Europe's largest employer. In **CHAPTER 9** Janet Martin covers some of the recent high profile healthcare incidents and the resultant changes to personnel management practice. Her chapter illustrates the wide-ranging impact upon the delivery of healthcare if personnel policies, staff recruitment, training, CPD programmes, resourcing and skill mix are not right. She explains how to establish and implement good standards in managing people.

Future editions of this book 1.14

Any publication that claims to cover the latest initiatives and current developments, will naturally be out of date, at least in some respects, the moment it is published. This is especially so for the subject matter of this publication as the entire arena of managing risk in healthcare is constantly changing. For the future it is planned that the publication will be regularly updated in successive editions and the guidance within the individual chapters expanded, so that healthcare organisations have continued access to up-to-the-minute, practical and quality advice.

Chapter 2
Managing Risk

This chapter covers:

- The concept and principles of risk management.

- The links between governance and risk management.

- Assessing risk, taking action and performance monitoring.

- Consequences of not managing risk.

- Risk, quality and assurance.

- Developing strategies to deal with risk.

Introduction   2.1

When confronted with a chapter on risk management, many readers may think it is a dull subject and, depending on how it is approached and discussed, it can be. However, risk management can be instructive, useful and instrumental in bringing about cultural change within an organisation. It can focus on the positive aspects in an organisation as opposed to negative ones, and it presents an excellent opportunity to bring about change as it allows professionals to challenge the way they think and behave.

Early in the 1990s, the Department of Health (DoH) risk management guidance tended to focus on estates, facilities, health, safety and disaster management, with very little aimed at clinical risk. For many healthcare professionals this was difficult to relate to in their daily work – the diagnosis, treatment and management of patients. The linkages between risk in clinical and non-clinical aspects of healthcare was not made at the time. Healthcare provision was not seen as an industry in its own right with a multitude of risk management issues to address. That has now changed. As we move through the 21st century, our knowledge and application of risk management to healthcare has matured, professionals now recognising that risk management applies to all aspects of a healthcare organisation, including clinical practice.

This chapter begins with an understanding of risk, followed by the building blocks needed to put an effective system of risk management in place. The chapter culminates with strategic development, which will allow practitioners and board directors to establish a workable framework for managing risk.

This chapter addresses the following issues:

- definitions and principles of risk management;
- the relationship of risk with governance and quality; and
- how risk management can be applied within the healthcare setting.

The aim is to give readers the ability to:

- define and understand the principles of risk management;
- identify, assess and control risks;
- understand how risk management fits with governance, controls and quality assurance;
- develop and introduce risk management into their organisation; and
- understand and accept the consequences of not managing risk.

Understanding risk and uncertainty   2.2

Although risk as a concept can be traced back to the early Greek civilizations, it is the Indo-Arabic numbering system and the use of mathematical probability 800 years ago that provided the basis for risk until the Renaissance period. It was then that risk emerged as a more serious subject concerned with forecasting the future through informed decision-making, an approach we still use today.

The early 20th century brought further development in risk through adoption of a scientific approach, first introduced by Willett[1] and later by Knight.[2] It is Knight's work that provides our basis for a classical approach to risk based on management science theory, observing that individuals have three key advantages in decision-making when it comes to risk. These are:

- knowledge of the problem itself;
- an understanding of the complete range of possible outcomes (measurable certainty); and
- the ability to objectively assess the likelihood of each outcome occurring.

Acquiring knowledge of a problem is reasonably straightforward, but understanding the range of possible outcomes is not, because of the introduction of uncertainty – the truly unforeseen. Measurable certainty is of course relevant, but in analysing risk, it is the implication of uncertainty that can cause the most disruption. A good example of this, especially in 20th century medicine, was the unforeseen damage to children as a result of thalidomide use during pregnancy. Whilst the maternal benefits were known, the risks to their children were not until they were born, resulting in the eventual withdrawal of thalidomide.

Knight also assumed that assessment of any likelihood (probability) is objective, when in fact it can be subjective. We must acknowledge that whilst risk and the management of risk is a science, it is not a perfect one in the sense that it is difficult, if not impossible, to separate risk from uncertainty. Risk management is therefore an imprecise science.

Bettis[3] took this abstract thinking about risk one step further and applied it to organisations. From this research, a distinction was drawn between using scientific models to determine risk, as opposed to those influenced by organisational behaviours where individual judgements become an important factor in determining risk. Once this subjectivity arises, uncertainty is inevitable.

Even in healthcare, it is the emphasis on trying to define and quantify risk in such a precise way that it becomes the end as opposed to a means to an end. That is not to say that determining risk and the probability of its outcome is not important – indeed health and safety legislation requires it – but it is only one part of risk management. This is an issue that will be revisited throughout the chapters of this book.

It is the understanding of risk and uncertainty that is crucial to addressing risk in healthcare, whether considered in relation to the organisation, the environment in which it operates, or the people involved or affected by it. A simple working definition of risk is proposed for use by readers as:

> 'the probability or likelihood that harm may occur, coupled with the consequences of that harm.'

Such harm could manifest itself in a number of ways, such as social exclusion, physical or psychological damage or financial impact, concepts which are alluded to in the chapters that follow, and in particular in **CHAPTER 6**.

Hazard versus risk   2.3

Before proceeding any futher, it is important, based on the definition proposed for users earlier, that there is an understanding of hazard so that a distinction can be drawn between hazard and risk.

Risk has been defined as the probability or likelihood that harm will occur and the consequences if it does. Hazard on the other hand is the ability to cause harm, the precursor to risk. For example, an electrical cord placed across a corridor is a hazard, while risk is the likelihood that someone would trip or fall as a result of it being placed there. By removing the cord, the hazard and the risk are eliminated. By covering the cord with a protective cover, the hazard is still present, but the risk is minimised. Definitions of hazard and risk have been developed more fully and over a long period of time within the field of occupational health and safety. **CHAPTER 6** deals more fully with these issues.

The first step, as shown in **TABLE 2.1**, is to consider the activities of an organisation – whether this is a precisely defined activity such as manual handling of equipment, or a wider activity such as surgery. Once the activity is identified, the next step is to identify hazards associated with the activity. Using surgery as the activity, some of the hazards identified are listed in **TABLE 2.1** along with their potential effects.

Table 2.1: Hazards in surgery

Hazard	Consequence
Anaesthetic equipment failure	Harm to or death of patient
Unmarked syringes	Wrong drug or dose given
Handling clinical waste	Cuts and exposure to biological agents
Needles	Exposure to biological agents
Slip, trip or fall	Injury to body
Use of disinfectants	Respiratory or skin sensitisation
Moving patient on to table	Back or shoulder injury
X-ray equipment	Over-exposure to radiation
Blood or body fluids	Exposure to biological agents

Principles of risk management   2.4

Put simply, risk management equates to good management practice; it therefore constitutes an overall management approach applicable to any organisation. Eight guiding principles can be used to develop a structured approach that will enable subsequent chapters to be set in context, with a background of essential skills in place.

Principles of risk management

(1)   A culture where risk management is considered an essential and positive element in the provision of healthcare.

(2)   Risk reduction and quality improvement are seen as activities worthy of being pursued.

(3)   Risk management often works within a statutory framework which cannot be ignored.

(4)   A risk management approach should provide a supportive structure for those involved in adverse incidents or errors by enabling a no-blame culture.

(5)   Processes should be strengthened and developed to allow for better identification of risk.

(6)   Managing risk is both a collective and an individual responsibility.

(7)   Recognise that resources may sometimes be required to address risk.

(8)   Every organisation should strive to understand the causes of risk, its link with quality and the consequences of failure.

Principle 1 – a culture where risk management is considered an essential and positive element in the provision of healthcare   2.5

Risk spans all functions in an organisation and should be seen as integral to both strategic and operational policy development. Healthcare professionals are more aware of the concept of risk and the importance that managing risk plays in the development and delivery of care than they were ten years ago. This awareness alone is not sufficient. Leaders within the organisation, from the board to clinicians, must drive risk management forward, provide a culture where lessons are learnt, blame is not apportioned and engender confidence in the open identification and resolution of risk is rewarded. This type of approach will ensure that important concerns do not get hidden because the culture of the organisation is such that it stifles staff speaking out rather than listening to them.

Principle 2 – risk reduction and quality improvement should be seen as activities worthy of being pursued   2.6

Many healthcare organisations are subject to review using internal and external review processes. For example, the Department of Health's Planning and Priorities Framework (PPF)[4], introduced in 2002–3 set public sector agreement targets for each NHS organisation. Royal College visits, Health and Safety Executive (HSE) inspections, National Audit Office (NAO) reviews and the Commission for Health Audit and Inspection (CHAI) conduct performance management exercises.

The National Institute of Clinical Excellence (NICE), DoH National Service Frameworks (NSFs) for conditions such as coronary heart disease, and the introduction of a Quality and Outcome Framework for general practitioners are performance management tools developed from a robust evidence base. Managing risk through a performance management framework is a route to improving quality. By focusing on quality improvement as a way of reducing risk may become much easier than perhaps originally envisaged if quality improvement is seen as one side of a coin, with risk reduction and management as the other.

Principle 3 – risk management often works within a statutory framework that cannot be ignored   2.7

A statutory framework is not confined to occupational health and safety. It embraces all aspects of the healthcare function and the duty of care owed by clinicians. By adopting a risk management approach, statutory obligations can be identified and fulfilled in a positive way, rather than as a means of avoiding litigation and prosecution.

Any risk management strategy should account for the extent to which education and development of staff is necessary so that they understand what is required of them from a statutory perspective, and thus are able to take responsibility for working within the law in its widest sense.

Principle 4 – a risk management approach should provide a supportive structure for those involved in adverse incidents or errors by enabling a no-blame culture 2.8

In the past, the NHS and other public bodies operated a culture of blame; this was evident in the language used and the way issues were approached when things went wrong. Many in the public sector have worked consistently over the years, and with some success, to overcome a negative culture by objectively looking at why an error or adverse event occurred, supporting staff and patients through the process and seeking improvements where possible. This has been based upon recognition that adverse events are most usually as a result of collective rather than individual error.

A good risk management approach looks beyond the negatives, overcomes the problems of professional boundaries and focuses on improving safety, processes and/or systems rather than seeking and allocating blame. This requires a cultural shift of some magnitude, coupled with sensitive handling. It should be seen as working within an ethical and legal framework aimed at getting the best out of individuals rather than penalising them when adverse events occur.

Principle 5 – processes should be strengthened and developed to allow for better identification of risk 2.9

Healthcare organisations are often described as data-rich, but information-poor. It is important not just to follow procedures by completing forms and writing reports for example, but to think about what this data suggests about how organisations and individuals are performing and, more importantly, the risks prevalent in healthcare and how they can be reduced.

Incident reports, patient complaints and suggestions, legal claims, morbidity and mortality data, audit results, risk assessments and research findings are sources of information. Often, however, they are not fully utilised to identify problems and improve practice. Much can be done to integrate information and make informed decisions about the risks in practice when information is utilised to its maximum potential. The introduction of a single unified electronic patient record will be a good tool for risk reduction, reducing the chances of information being held elsewhere, and therefore not accessible, often to the detriment of the patient.

Principle 6 – managing risk is both a collective and an individual responsibility 2.10

People often say 'they should do something', by which they mean the organisation. But in fact the organisation is a collective of individuals working towards the development and delivery of healthcare. In many cases this phrase is targeted at board members aimed at placing decision-making with them in order to allocate responsibility for perceived or actual failures. It has to be recognised that there is individual as well as collective responsibility and this sense of ownership needs to be accounted for in the way an organisation approaches and introduces risk management. Whilst there is corporate responsibility, each individual also has a responsibility in law, and arguably morally, to identify risk and take steps to control it within healthcare.

Principle 7 – recognise that resources may sometimes be required to address risk 2.11

It is unrealistic and naïve to think that all risk can be reduced without some investment, whether in the form of human resource or finances. In many instances the financial implications will be limited as working differently may be all that is required.

Notwithstanding financial constraints or lack of human resources – particularly for safety matters – is not a defence in law to ignore risk. On the other hand, it does not make economic sense, either in the public or private sector, to be reckless with money to reduce every identified risk, irrespective of the extent of the risk identified. To counter this and retain a sense of pragmatism, it is important to determine what risks are acceptable and what risks are not, often done through a process of risk prioritisation. This cannot be done in isolation, but in an environment of openness and inclusivity.

Principle 8 – every organisation should strive to understand the causes of risk, its link with quality and the consequences of failure 2.12

Risk management is a learning process reliant on methods to identify, assess and control risk. It has to form part of other approaches used by clinicians, staff and managers on a day-to-day basis.

Causes of risk may stem from the way the organisation is structured, the number of staff employed and their mix of skills, or from an absence of guidance or procedures, which set out what is expected of staff. Risk may be linked to the physical or psychological environment, to behaviour, competency or levels of supervision. Using a model to educate individuals on the links between risk and quality is beneficial, giving people the skills and competencies they need to manage both areas.

13

Eight principles have been outlined, each with a summary of the issues that need to be considered and which should form part of an overall strategy for risk management, discussed later in this chapter.

The process of risk management   2.13

Risk management is about the planning, organisation and direction of a programme that will identify, assess and ultimately control risk. It offers a framework which others can work to and operate within. The best way to illustrate this is shown in **FIGURE 2.1**.

Figure 2.1: The risk management process

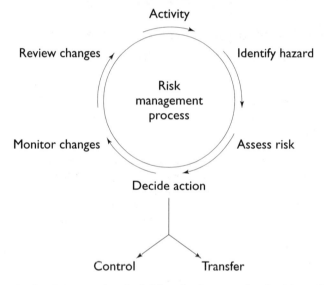

Every organisation has some level of risk, whether associated with medical treatment, financial planning, or the recruitment and retention of staff. Risk management brings the risks from these activities together in order to allow them to be viewed both strategically and operationally. This in turn will allow decision-makers to consider the quantity and extent of risk presented and to make choices about managing them.

The interdependency of risk   2.14

Risk can be categorised in a number of ways and not unusually in healthcare into clinical or non-clinical categories. For example, clinical incidents may also have health and safety ramifications for individual staff. Faulty x-ray equipment may deliver an inappropriate dose to the patient and may also result in staff over-exposure. It is important to understand the interdependency and effect different types of risk may have on each other.

Consider the recent increase in revenue to the NHS through taxation, as a result of government policy. This has provided an opportunity to increase and enhance clinical services for patients, in essence reducing some element of risk around access to services. However, inflationary pressures may in fact take up such a percentage of the new investment that as a result, the reduction in risk may not be as great as originally thought.

Research and clinical evidence may on the one hand identify how to reduce risk for one disease, but increase the risk of another occurring. The most obvious case is in the use of cytotoxic drugs to treat cancer.

Assessing risk   2.15

Identifying hazards can be relatively straightforward. It is determining whether a risk exists, and if so to what extent, that can be the most problematic. It is the stage where human factors come into play because of the subjectivity a person will bring to the assessment process, even if a quantitative approach is applied. The assessment process entails analysing the hazard and determining, based on the information and evidence available, the extent of the risk and actions to reduce risk. This is covered in more detail through a number of different chapters, but for the purposes of setting the strategic context, an overview of some of the features of risk assessment are provided below.

Quantitative versus qualitative approaches   2.16

Quantitative and/or qualitative methodologies are equally applicable when assessing risk. Either way, there is no right or wrong answer, nor should the conclusions be seen as forever binding, but rather taken as a snapshot of what the level of risk appears to be at that point of time.

The extent of risk can be a moving target and is underpinned by a degree of uncertainty as previously discussed. FIGURE 2.2 illustrates a relatively simplistic approach to determining the level or extent of risk, using two parameters: probability and impact. Other assessment models include frequency as a third parameter. Notwithstanding the complexities that arise with the model used, the generic approach outlined gives a useful assessment. The next step is to minimise or, in some cases, eliminate risk.

Figure 2.2: Probability and impact of risk

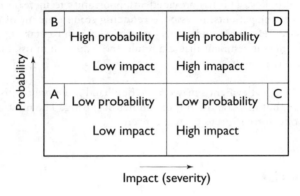

Impact (severity)

Transfer or control?   2.17

In **FIGURE 2.1** two paths can be taken – either controlling or transferring risk. The majority of healthcare providers will usually control risk as opposed to transferring it although the thinking around this is changing. For example, contracting out services is one way to transfer risk, putting the responsibility with others rather than the organisation itself. This will of course be dependent on the circumstances, the level of risk exposure and whether it is feasible, morally and economically to transfer risk.

One example where risk is transferred is via the private finance initiative (PFI), although even with this, NHS trusts do carry risk, financial as well as those related to employment. Risk management issues in connection with PFI are dealt with in **CHAPTER 3** and **CHAPTER 7**. Another example is the commissioning of day surgery from independent providers, transferring risk from NHS organisations and establishing legally binding contracts which require the provider to manage clinical and non-clinical risk.

A third element is coming more to the fore – risk sharing. This has become apparent with the primary care trusts (PCTs) as they mature within the NHS. Risks are now being shared amongst a number of PCTs in their role as commissioners, allowing a more flexible and manageable approach to financial management, particularly in areas where demand for services cannot be predicted with a level of confidence (e.g. individual packages of care, free nursing care). With the introduction of patient choice, where patients can choose the type of treatment and the mode of delivery including where it may be delivered, risk sharing will play a much more important role within the NHS.

The language of risk   2.18

It is important to consider how risk is expressed. Use of words such as 'high' and 'low' in assessments, may suggest the seriousness or otherwise of the risk. Other possible expressions used include 'minor', 'major', 'critical', 'untoward', 'serious' and the like. These words are open to interpretation, but are however useful in order to rank and prioritise risk.

In everyday use, precise definitions of risk may be irrelevant because general concepts are understood. However, when an incident does occur, the lack of a universally understood term can create problems within an organisation, initiating reactions and behaviours that in hindsight may have been misplaced. The opposite is also true. The language we use can act as a distraction from risks that are truly significant, with great effort applied to issues which are of little significance. It is important that when we come to developing a risk management strategy later in this chapter, we have an understanding of what specific terms mean and how they should be used (see **2.43** **DEFINING RISK AND EXPRESSIONS OF RISK**).

Monitoring and reviewing   2.19

Deciding what is the best course of action is by far the most difficult because of the uncertainty that may surround the decision. It is important that irrespective of what action is taken, the way the decision was made and the process used to inform it are transparent and understood.

Once a decision is taken about, whether to transfer, control or share risk, the implementation of the decision should always be monitored. This is good management practice and fits in with the concept of assuring the quality of the process followed.

Taking a decision on risk control cannot be done in isolation, but must be considered within the context of what is happening elsewhere in the organisation. Reducing risk in one situation may increase risks in other areas.

Organisation, environment, the person   2.20

There are three areas that should be borne in mind when monitoring changes. These will feature in the development of a risk management strategy. They are:

- **Organisation**: financial management, organisational structure, legal requirements, standards, culture, priorities and both external and internal influences.

- **Environment**: support, workload, physical and psychological environments.

- **Person**:
  - ○   if a patient: the nature and complexity of their condition, communication skills and social factors;
  - ○   if an employee: their knowledge, skills, competency and mental health; and

    ○   if a visitor: their expectations and their unfamiliarity with where they are.

This is illustrated in **FIGURE 2.3**

Figure 2.3: Risk in context

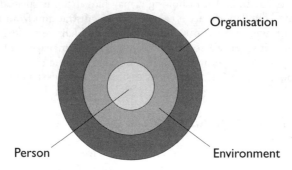

It can be inferred from **FIGURE 2.3** that problems exhibited within the organisation will eventually have an impact individuals. Get the organisation right, and the risks can be minimised for others.

Consequences of not managing risk   2.21

The worst consequence of not managing risk could be the loss of life or lives. This could involve a patient undergoing treatment or employees undertaking their daily duties. Readers will recall news stories where employees have been killed or severely injured in the construction industry or through other industrial processes, or where patients have received the wrong or inappropriate treatment. Investigations of these tragic events usually identify weaknesses in the identification, management and control of risk.

The outcome of such investigations seen over the past few years in healthcare illustrates this point. The word 'Bristol' stirs memories of the children's heart surgery scandal (**SEE KEY REFERENCES, APPENDIX 1**) and 'Shipman' the deaths of many elderly people cared for by a general practitioner in primary care. The outcome of the enquiries still overshadows the good clinical care that is provided on a daily basis within the NHS. One consequence, therefore, of not managing risk is the damage to an organisation's or indeed whole institution's, reputation and the associated lack of public confidence in future use of the services provided by the organisation.

Costs to the organisation   2.22

Repeatedly the behaviour exhibited by individuals and organisations such as shortcuts in systems and processes, a deliberate lack of investment in key functional areas, denying training opportunities to staff, culminates in some damage. More recently the prosecution of individuals or corporate bodies is a public signal that poor risk management will not be tolerated. For the first time doctors have been prosecuted for errors in treatment. Organisations will have to manage this, avoiding the reaction to hide or not disclose errors that have been made to avoid disclosure, which may lead to prosecution. This balance is an important one, on which the board and senior clinicians in the NHS must provide leadership.

Another consequence of an organisation not managing risk is increased costs, as illustrated in the box below. From an assurance perspective, boards must be satisfied that through the application of risk management, the costs to the organisation need to be quantified in order for it to make an informed decision about how to manage risks. The use of organisational registers, as required through the Department of Health's controls assurance framework, is an aid to this process, but will not provide the whole picture. Costs to the organisation, which may be predominately financially focused, will need to account for public and patient confidence, something on which a cost can not be assigned.

Risk and the law   2.23

There is recourse to the law for those who want retribution for what has happened to them. This is an individual's right and should not be feared. The increased projected costs of clinical negligence claims year on year in the UK point to a society that is more willing to seek compensation through the courts if dissatisfied. It also points to a lack of public confidence that public sector bodies, such as the NHS, are open and honest in what they do and how they manage risks associated with their activities.

A defensive approach   2.24

Whilst this trend is not as commonplace as in the United States, it is a worry nonetheless. The tendency for organisations, particularly healthcare providers, is to become defensive in their practice, in essence withdrawing to protect the organisation as a whole. This defensive approach pushes risk management into a function that is seen by the public as a way to protect doctors and nurses from litigation, rather than as a method by which to highlight and improve care. The Clinical Negligence Scheme for Trusts (CNST), despite its efforts to be seen as a positive force for good, is publicly committed to reducing the cost of litigation by employing risk management methods. This approach has led many in the healthcare field to see these standards as simply an exercise in protecting a hospital or primary care trust rather than how they should be viewed – standards aimed at improving the quality of care provided.

Nonetheless, the cost of litigation is increasing as a more consumer-driven society develops. The consequence to NHS trusts, including those in primary care, and independent practitioners is an increase in the insurance premium required to cover potential liabilities. For a large hospital, this can be quite substantive. It is also lost money, taken out of clinical care and held to offset the unforeseen, but not the unforeseeable.

The introduction of patient choice, where patients can choose where they wish to be treated and by whom, will mean that each NHS organisation will have to provide the same high standards of care and to publish their clinical outcomes and complication rates. One could speculate that hospitals or primary care trusts that have a high number of complaints and/or litigation cases will not be seen as the preferred provider of care by patients.

Two examples of poorly managed risk

Poor infection control management

A hospital-acquired infection is diagnosed in a ward. Infection control measures have been developed, but are not followed by nursing and medical staff. As a result, the infection spreads and patients with a higher risk of infection due to their medical condition become infected. Because the organism is resistant to normally prescribed antibiotics, patients have to be treated with different intravenous antibiotics, presenting them with additional risks and incurring higher costs to the organisation. The length of stay at the hospital for these patients may be increased, resulting in a lack of beds for other patients.

Poor employee relations

One community service within a primary care trust has a higher than average sickness/absence rate plus a number of unfilled vacancies despite a good rate of pay and no national shortage of trained staff in this field. A review of recruitment and retention information shows a higher than average turnover in staff. Anecdotal evidence suggests that the manager of the service has poor communication skills, does not delegate to others, refuses staff training and development and is quite difficult to work with. As a result, potential employees in the market will not apply for jobs, seeking employment at the neighbouring trust instead. The consequence of this is a demoralised workforce for those who remain and a less than adequate service because of staff vacancies. To counter this, agency staff would need to be employed to ensure safe staffing levels – a financial drain on the service's budget – in addition to covering those who are sick or otherwise absent.

Risk and quality   2.25

One of the most important aspects of risk is to consider its link with quality, because of the close alignment of the principles of quality assurance and risk management. It can be said that risk and quality are interchangeable as intiatives to reduce risk can lead to improved quality and vice versa. TABLE 2.2 below describes how the two management systems relate.

Table 2.2: Quality assurance and risk management

Quality assurance	Risk management
Establish organisational goals Assess proce dures in place to achieve goals of the service or activity	Identify risks associated with activity Assess risk as it affects all elements of the service or activity
Implement actions and measures to overcome problems	Develop and implement control measures to reduce risks
Monitor to assure desired result has been achieved	Monitor changes to ensure risks have been minimised
Document effectiveness of changes	Document effectiveness of changes

One of the simplest ways of differentiating quality assurance from risk management is to think of quality measures as the outcome of a process, whereas risk management will concentrate on the input to a process, as illustrated in **FIGURE 2.4**.

Figure 2.4: Risk and quality

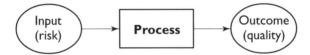

The discerning will see fault with this simple theory, noting that there are many assumptions inherent in this model, the first being that the risk is identified, known and without uncertainty and that using risk as the input, the outcome will be improved quality. How quality is measured and whether perception is enough, particularly if it improves morale amongst staff or engenders a sense of confidence by the public is a question that has yet to be answered.

Governance and risk management 2.26

A series of major corporate failures in the UK and USA lead to a number of reports aimed at improving corporate business processes and acountability. One of these, the *Turnbull Report* (SEE KEY REFERENCES, APPENDIX 1) required the identification of significant risks faced by an organisation. The findings are just as relevant to the NHS as they are to those companies listed on the London Stock Exchange.

From this report sprang clinical governance – taking the same concepts and applying them within a clinical setting – again in order to ensure there was transparency in the way healthcare was organised and operated and, importantly, to make sure that the public could scrutinise how the public sector operates. Two Department of Health policy statements in the late 1990s, *The New NHS: Modern, Dependable* and *A First Class Service* and more recently, the Government's report on the NHS, as produced by the Treasury Department, known as the *Wanless Report*[5], outline the importance of quality and risk management and the need to have a governance framework to deliver improvements in health services.

In 2002, the NHS issued guidance entitled *Assurance – The Board Agenda*[6] (see **KEY REFERENCES, APPENDIX 1**), asking each organisation to ensure that it was confident in how systems, policies and people were operating that could demonstrate effectiveness, accounted for key risks and established a risk management framework that facilitated, not hindered, performance. The following year the NHS Appointments Commission issued guidance on governing in the NHS[7]. This is a 'must read' for board level directors, senior managers and clinical leaders in the NHS. It sets out the principles for a strong system of governance and introduces, for the first time, the concept of integrated governance, bringing together the facets of clinical and corporate governance into a framework that, if operated well, will address the breadth of risk issues within an organisation. The guidance outlines the Governance Framework:

- strategic planning and objective setting;

- using systems to ensure objectives are met such as clinical governance, risk management systems and financial management systems; and

- ensuring systems themselves embody satisfactory controls – controls assurance.

Corporate responsibility is discussed, stressing accountability and responsibility and the importance of three public service values: accountability, probity and openness. These are drawn together in core standards of care, expressed as a Code of Conduct for NHS Managers as (see **KEY REFERENCES, APPENDIX 1**):

- making the care and safety of patients the first concern and acting to protect them from risk

- respecting the public, patients, relatives, carers, NHS staff and partners in other agencies

- being honest and acting with integrity

- accepting responsibility for work and the proper performance of people being managed

- showing commitment to working as a team member by working with NHS colleagues and the wider community

- taking responsibility for personal learning and development

The first core standard refers to protecting patients from risk, further emphasising the importance of risk management in the NHS, strategically and operationally, as a collective as well as individuals. Integrated governance is the high level, strategic overview of issues, but as seen, it must be supported by the detailed work undertaken through a range of methods such as controls assurance, regulatory and clinical governance reviews and audits.

Controls assurance 2.27

Controls assurance was first introduced in the NHS in 1999. This process, originally introduced for financial management, has now been extended to many of the functions of healthcare and is used to ensure there is a system for the effective control of risk. NHS organisation are required to publish a *Statement of Internal Control*[8], which indicates how the public can be assured that the organisation does identify, manage and control its risks.

Risk management is seen as the glue that binds the functions of financial management, the care environment and clinical practice together (see **FIGURE 2.5**). It is itself a function that can be applied to the financial setting, how the environment is organised and to how clinical care is delivered. The latter subject is discussed in more depth in **CHAPTER 4**.

Each of the controls assurance standards has a number of compliance criteria. The core risk management standard looks at the capability within the organisation, the strategy and how it is implemented, what training and communication mechanisms are in place and, lastly, how a risk management strategy is monitored and evaluated. The standards can be found on the Controls Assurance website: www.controlsassurance.gov.uk which will give much more in-depth information about controls assurance requirements. The Controls Assurance Support Unit (CASU) at Keele University, established by the Department of Health, can also be contacted. They will assist NHS organisations to improve risk management and ultimately the quality of services provided in the NHS.

Figure 2.5: Controls assurance (source: NHS Executive (see KEY REFER-ENCES, APPENDIX 1))

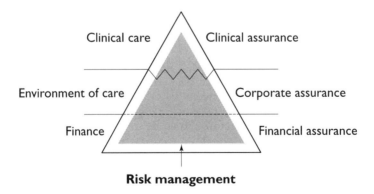

Developing a risk management strategy 2.28

Developing a risk management strategy in many respects is easy as it is simply articulating, often on paper, the vision of an organisation about how it will manage risk. What is not so easy is effectively changing the way the organisation perceives and deals with risk, despite the assurances that may be put in place. That is the real challenge.

When developing any type of strategy, there are a number of steps to be undertaken: analysing what currently goes on in the organisation regarding risk management, followed by a critical analysis of gaps or improvements required (gap analysis), and culminating in a strategic direction with clear aims and objectives.

Resources 2.29

During strategic development, resources are required, not necessarily in financial terms, but in terms of the people and time needed to develop and crucially, implement a comprehensive, all-embracing risk management strategy. In this regard, the strategy should reflect the breadth of risk, encompassing clinical as well as non-clinical issues such as health and safety, organisational and legal issues. All of these should be accounted for so that the strategy is clear, concise and comprehensive.

Risk management may require additional financial resources that will need to be accounted for. The arguments run parallel with introducing quality systems into an organisation where some investment may be required up front, but the gains at the end of the process are significantly higher than the original outlay. Risk management is often cost effective over time. Decisions to be taken on investment should include a cost benefit analysis of whether to invest or not, judged against potential consequences will be a key feature of any discussion on future investment.

A positive process 2.30

The biggest opportunity and challenge to introducing a risk management strategy is gaining the hearts and minds of those in the organisation, to embrace and effect change. Risk management therefore should be seen as a positive process, not a punitive one. It should foster a focus on learning, not blame. There should be tangible outcomes for staff and patients to see – better clinical outcomes, an improved work environment and/or reduced stress levels for staff and patients alike.

Purpose of the strategy 2.31

The purpose of a strategy is to determine the direction an organisation should be heading towards. In order to do this, three key elements must be in place:

- strategic analysis (where are we now);

- strategic choice (where do we want to be); and

- strategic implementation (how do we get there).

The corporate strategy model shown in **FIGURE 2.6** can be used to help develop a risk management strategy.

Strategic analysis entails much of what was discussed earlier, so that an understanding is created of the political, economic and social environment in which healthcare operates. Whether it is general practice, a hospital or community setting, there will be a number of internal and external influences to account for, such as legislation and Department of Health guidance. The introduction of new controls assurance standards is an example of this. In addition, the healthcare organisation will need to look at the people, systems and resources that are in place to deliver its aims.

Figure 2.6: A corporate strategy model[9]

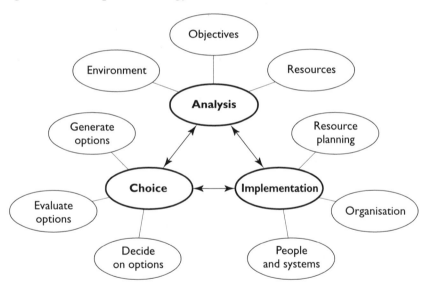

Strategic analysis – where are we now?

Objectives   2.32

The review of where an organisation is in terms of risk management is the first step in developing a risk management strategy. The purpose is to minimise and, if possible, eliminate risks to the organisation, the environment and people who may be affected (See **FIGURE 2.3**). The expectations and objectives in place will, set the direction for the future.

Environment 2.33

Internal and external influences imposed upon and operating within the organisation will need to be accounted for as part of the environmental evaluation. It is necessary to be aware of, and sensitive to, what influences are about, taking account of them, but being mindful of the 'must-do's' placed on an organisation. The Public Sector Agreement (PSA) targets in the DoH's Planning and Priorities Framework (PPF) and the continued publication of national service frameworks (NSFs) are two good examples – the risk of not meeting their requirements or quality standards would have a significant impact on a NHS organisation, presenting an organisation risk in its own right.

Resources 2.34

The third component of strategic analysis should look at both financial and human resource. Who, for example, is going to lead the risk management process – at board level, at directorate level and within clinical and non-clinical services? Will the approach taken be based on everyone accepting responsibility for managing risk and in so doing, who will provide the leadership to drive the process forward? Trying to develop a risk management strategy without the resources needed will end in confusion and a job half done, and people not believing in the value of the work they have completed. The converse however is building up an industry in its own right where it drives itself, consumes resources, is seen as separate from the operational management of risk and worst of all, allows people to think that risk management is 'their job', thus losing the individual responsibility one is trying to foster.

Strategic choice: where do we want to be?

Generate options 2.35

Generating options can often be challenging and exciting, allowing people to express their ideas about how things can be done differently. Involving people is vitally important because it generates the best ideas, and instils a sense of worth, ownership and commitment in the process.

This does not mean everyone in the organisation has to be involved however desirable, but it should include, as a minimum, those people who have an understanding of the issues and of what could be done. This should encompass people from a range of professional groups, such as nurses, doctors, therapists, managers, technicians, maintenance, administrative and clerical staff. Together they should formulate a series of options. Workshops, task groups, open meetings or small groups working by speciality are a few ways that this can be achieved. The more involvement there is, the easier it is to gain ownership of the strategy as it emerges.

Evaluate options   2.36

Once options for a strategic approach to risk have been identified, evaluating options is the next step. This lends credibility to the process and sets the ideas generated into a realistic framework. This needs to be handled skilfully and with sensitivity, for once others are engaged in the process, it is detrimental to then disillusion and isolate them through an evaluation process.

To avoid this, involve others in determining the criteria used to evaluate the options generated. For example, options might be generated ranging from doing nothing, to one option where committees and groups are established to work on specific risk issues. Criteria developed and applied to these options could include the amount of resources needed and whether the option generated delivers the best value for the organisation. Even by applying this or any other criteria, subjectivity arises and rightly so. It will need to be challenged in order to reach a position where decisions are more robust. As long as everyone is clear how options and how decisions are made, then the process of evaluation will stand up to any scrutiny.

Strategic implementation – how do we get there?   2.37

Once the choices have been presented and a decision made about a risk management approach, strategic development and implementation follows. To do this, three elements, need to be considered:

- how the organisation is structured;
- what people and systems are in place and; and
- what resources and planning is required to put the strategy into place.

A time element should accompany this stage of the process for it cannot all be done at once, but should be staged and evaluated as the implementation unfolds.

Structure and culture of the organisation   2.38

The structure and importantly the culture of the organisation are an issue for anyone introducing a risk management strategy. Much of this concerns understanding collective and individual responsibilities in the organisation and what the lines of accountability are.

Risk management is everyone's responsibility. One only has to look to legislation or codes of professional conduct to see this. It is how the levels of responsibility are delineated that takes centre stage. For example, a nurse will be expected to identify, assess and control where possible risks to patients, the environment and staff. However, the nurse may not be in a position to solely control the risk because it may require additional resource over which they do not have authority.

That does not negate the nurse's responsibility, but it does highlight the importance of setting out clear levels of accountability and responsibility and where decision-making lies.

People and systems   2.39

A chief executive in the NHS, as an accountable officer to the board, has the ultimate responsibility for risk management. The board is responsible for assuring itself and thus the public, that it is confident in the systems, processes and people in place that risks are identified and managed. Implementation is delegated on a day-to-day basis to others within the organisation who are equipped to introduce a risk management strategy in a way that is inclusive, driven by those who provide care and that ultimately leads to changes.

Clinicians and managers discharge their operational duties through the implementation of policies, procedures, guidance and protocols. It is the type of organisational rules that help bind an organisation into a structure that performs. Risk management is no different. Employees' responsibilities lie in working to the organisational rules and maintaining their awareness of how they can influence and make a difference. This is the real change agent for managing risk.

Risk management strategy in practice   2.40

Thus far the corporate strategy model has been used to illustrate the process of setting about a strategy for risk management, but this has been confined to discussions based on models and theory rather than what really happens in practice. So how is a risk management strategy developed and introduced?

One way forward is for a group of individuals led by a senior manager and clinician to undertake the work as outlined in the corporate strategy model in **FIGURE 2.6**, in order to gain an understanding of how to set about introducing change within the organisation. There are six important ingredients that are required for a risk management strategy, even in its early development. These ingredients will set the tone of the strategy document and indicate how it will be introduced. These are:

Elements of a risk management strategy

(1) Having the support of the board.

(2) Writing a strategy that is understandable.

(3) Defining risk and associated terminology.

(4) Learning.

(5) Communication.

(6) Tools of the trade.

---

(1) Having the support of the board 2.41

It is nearly impossible to successfully introduce risk management into an organisation without the full support of the board; the chairperson, chief executive, directors and non-executive directors. Because they are the ultimate decision-makers, if their support is not forthcoming, any risk management strategy will fail, no matter how good it is.

Therefore it must be developed with the visible and undeniable support of the board. Assurance and inspection bodies are looking for a signature by the chief executive to a policy or strategy document as well as formal acceptance of it at board level. In addition, they will look for it to be effectively communicated so that staff and members of the public are aware of the organisation's commitment to managing risk.

There should be an appointed executive director with responsibility at board level for ensuring a strategy is developed and in place. Often a non-executive director will take a scrutiny role. This will however vary, according to the structure of the healthcare organisation. For example, in a large teaching hospital, the medical director or director of nursing will typically take the lead, usually as part of clinical governance. In a primary care trust, the lead may be one of the directors or alternatively the clinical governance lead. Irrespective of the type of healthcare organisation, there needs to be a named senior person who will voice issues at board level and provide leadership and support to others on behalf of the chief executive and senior management team.

(2) Writing a strategy that is understandable 2.42

Strategy documents can be written in two parts, the background to the strategy and objectives, supported by a policy that sets out the operational procedures required to deliver the objectives. In this way a strategy can be confined to a few pages, with the policy and subsequent procedures providing the basis and detail respectively. The strategy sets the direction of travel, the policy outlines how the journey will be made, assigning responsibility in the delivery, and the procedures provide detailed instructions for each part of the journey.

A strategy should be written in plain language and accessible to those whose first language is not English or who have a disability, so that stakeholders can understand what its intentions are and, more importantly, how these intentions are to be implemented. In this regard, it is useful to have non-executive directors or members of the public involved in its construction to avoid the use of unintelligible management and clinical jargon.

A strategy should be realistic. It should make some allowance for scanning the horizon for what is expected now and in the future. The strategy will provide a basis for short-term changes as well as longer-term ones, say over three to five years. Strategic documents should be subject to review with an acknowledgement that things may change due to external factors, but the essence of what is being achieved – reducing risk – will not.

(3) Defining risk and expressions of risk 2.43

The document should provide a working definition of risk. It should also give some guidance as to how terminology should be used and what it means. It is preferable to work to common definitions used by others such as the DoH for consistency and this should be stated somewhere at the outset of a strategic document.

(4) Learning 2.44

The strategy should explain the philosophy of the organisation, its culture and how learning will be used to improve the quality of care and the reduction of risk. This is really about making sure the blame culture, if present, is eventually eliminated and, where it has been eliminated, to make sure it does not re-emerge.

Any good risk management programme should encompass learning as the platform from which to achieve its full potential. By adopting this approach, the strategy should include teaching and training as a key element of the programme plus an effective communication plan that supports the whole of the strategy.

The strategy, will include an appraisal and personal development plan. In other words, each individual's responsibility in the management of risk should be part of their regular performance appraisal. Milestones for achievement, dependent on the job in the organisation, should be included. By using appraisal as a route map for learning, evaluation and changes in practice can happen in an informative and proactive way.

For clinical staff, one way of introducing risk management into their practice would be to assess, as part of their appraisal, how many clinical events they reported against the number of consultations as well as the outcome of the events reported. It is the outcomes that are most important; addressing these ensures there is involvement of clinicians in addressing risk and quality issues.

(5) Communication 2.45

Communication forms an important part of the strategy document. For instance, what mechanisms will be used to communicate with staff, patients and the public about what needs to be done? It is unwise to invent complex mechanisms for selling the message. It is far better to use successful, tried and tested ones, exploring what methods of communication people are most likely to use.

Electronic communications systems   **2.46**

With an increased reliance on electronic communication systems in the NHS, one of the best communication tools is email for key messages, supported by an intranet site that allows staff to find out what is happening and access websites for further information and learning. For example, the risk management strategy can be loaded on an intranet with hyperlinks to the DoH controls assurance website. Another, more innovative example is using clinical information systems such as pathology results electronic reporting, and presenting risk information through that medium. This can instil a sense of risk management with young clinicians who will be the people to take forward risk management in the future. To educate them as they progress through an organisation is one of the most enduring and successful communication strategies to apply. The introduction of a single unified patient record in the coming years will give ample opportunity for developing ways of identifying clinical risks, one that should be harnessed and exploited to its full potential.

Whatever communication systems are used, their effectiveness must be evaluated. There is little value in using a staff newsletter to relate vital information if it is not read.

(6) Tools of the trade   **2.47**

Lastly, a strategy should set the direction for implementation, normally by giving staff a toolkit of ideas and guidance on how to proceed. For instance, the strategy might state that the tools needed to identify, assess and control risk are:

• incident reports;

• complaints and claims information;

• morbidity and mortality data;

• clinical and non-clinical audit information;

• risk assessments; and

• external reports from, for example, the NAO, HSE, CHAI, CNST and auditors.

The strategy should also establish the links between these tools and how the information will be used. Granted, some of this level of detail is more appropriate for procedure documents, but some indication of what is required to deliver change is necessary. It could simply be a statement in the strategy document that says: 'Risk assessment will be used to determine the extent of risk, supported by information from a number of sources, such as incident report data.'

Successful implementation   2.48

In summary, producing a risk management strategy can be straightforward provided the ingredients as listed are in place. However, do not underestimate the scale of the task in implementing a risk management strategy. The most important ingredient is communication. If the right message is given about what the strategy is, especially at board level, and it is backed up with learning, then the tools of the trade will fall into place. Make sure the support is there from the board from the onset and, over time, the strategy, its aims and objectives will be achieved.

A leading approach to managing risk   2.49

As this chapter makes clear, a number of consequences can arise if risk management is not developed and introduced, and an organisation and its people can be exposed to damage of whatever magnitude. It is only through leadership, constant communication and demonstration (e.g. leading by example) that managing risk will benefit all. This benefit can show up in increased productivity and a more confident and efficient workforce.

There is also a stark reality for those who take on the mantle of risk management and lead it in their organisation, and that is that this subject competes with many other pressing priorities in a fast-paced world. This is particularly true within the healthcare sector and it cannot be ignored. By embracing risk management as part of the foundation and making it part of everyday language, this can be overcome.

This chapter goes some way to outlining a way forward for those wishing to embark on this journey, a journey which is well worth taking. Success lies in making risk management an integral part of the daily business of healthcare, not an additional bureaucratic burden aimed at preventing claims or seen as an imposition from above. It takes leadership, backed up by sound communication and negotiation skills by those involved. If these are applied, an organisation secure in how it operates, with a view of risk as a positive approach to improving practice, will emerge.

References

See also KEY REFERENCES, Appendix 1
1   Willett, AH (1951), *The Economic Theory of Risk and Insurance*, Irwin Publishers, Illinois, USA.
2   Knight, TH (1921), *Risk, Uncertainty and Profit*, Houghton Mifflin Company, New York, USA.
3   Bettis, RA (1982) 'Risk considerations in modelling corporate strategy', *Academy of Management Proceedings*, New York, USA.
4   Department of Health (2002) *Planning and Priorities Framework*, Department of Health, UK
5   Department of the Treasury (2002) *The Wanless Report*, Department of the Treasury, UK
6   Department of Health (2003) *Assurance: the Board Agenda*, Department of Health, UK

7 Department of Health (2003) *Governing the NHS – A guide for NHS Boards*, Department of Health, UK
8 Department of Health (2003) *Statement of Internal Control*, Chief Executive Bulletin November 2003, Department of Health, UK
9 Adapted from the work of Johnson, G and Scholes, K (1989) *Exploring Corporate Strategy*, Prentice Hall Publishers, Hertfordshire.

Further information

Berstein, PL (1996) *Against the Gods: The Remarkable Story of Risk*, John Wiley and Sons, New York, 1996.

Burrows, M (2000) 'Trauma care, a team approach', *Risk Management*, Butterworth Heinemann, Oxford.

Burrows, M (1994) *Risk Management Applications in Healthcare*, dissertation submitted to Leicester University.

Burrows, M (2000) *Consent to Treatment,* dissertation submitted to Cardiff University.

Carter, RL (1994) *Handbook of Risk Management*, Kluwer Publishing, Surrey.

Collis, D (1992) 'The Strategic Management of Uncertainty' *European Management Journal*, Vol 10, no 2, pp125–135.

Rockett, JP (1999) 'Definitions are not what they seem', *Risk Management, An International Journal*, Vol 1, no 3.

Rowe, WD (1977) *Anatomy of Risk*, Wiley Publishers, New York.

Wilson, C (1987) *Quality Assurance and Risk Management: Two sides of the same coin*, unpublished paper, Canadian Institute of Law and Medicine Fall Conference, Toronto.

Stalvies, C (2000) 'Taking a risk – and managing it', *Health Care Risk Report*, Vol 6, no 9, pp18–19.

Useful websites

www.controlsassurance.gov.uk

www.doh.gov.uk

www.nhsla.gov.uk

Chapter 3
Managing Organisational Change

This chapter covers:

- Models of organisational change and how they help manage risk.

- The role of project management.

- Drivers for change within the NHS.

- Risks of organisational change.

- Legal framework.

- The Private Finance Initiative.

- Learning from organisational change – trust mergers, PCGs and PCTs, Shared Services, Shifting the Balance of Power, Foundation and Care trusts.

- The medical workforce change agenda – the consultant contract, GMS contract, doctors working hours.

Introduction   3.1

The NHS is permanently affected by change and this impacts upon risk in a major way. Whether organisational change is at a strategic or front-line level, there is always the need to ensure there are no gaps in service provision, and that service provision continues and is safe. In addition, the imperative to provide 'seamless care' for patients means that change for many frontline managers involves whole systems thinking – tackling complex, interdependent systems, in a collective way.

This chapter aims to provide a practical approach, as opposed to an academic review, to managing organisational change in the healthcare setting, drawing on lessons from past reorganisations and restructuring. It focuses primarily on the people management aspects, but not exclusively, and reviews some of the current change agenda issues and ramifications for the wider health and social care community.

Models of organisational change – how they help us identify risk   3.2

The report *Managing change in the NHS – organisational change*[1] reviews the litera-ture on change management and the evidence base for the different theoretical approaches. The review examines what is meant by change in the NHS context, and the value or extent of use of different academic models. Many of the approaches in the literature assume change can be rational and orderly, while in practice it is often chaotic, with shifting goals and unexpected outcomes.

This is seen in some of the examples outlined later in this chapter, where addi-tional factors are often added to the equation of change, or success in one change programme affects the achievement of other goals.

The NHS is affected by many issues which lead to the need for organisational change. Examples include:

* Government targets and priorities.

* Multiple stakeholders.

* Changing technologies.

* Mutual role dependence.

* Professional autonomy of many staff.

Examining the current and past change programmes supports the view that the NHS is an organisation subject to challenges and constraints arising from these characteristics, but also subject to continuous, emergent or seeming unplanned change.

The best change models and tools are therefore those which help us to understand:

* The nature and extent of the change programme.

* Deadlines for achievement.

* Identification of programme outcomes.

* How risk may arise.

* Identification of risk management strategies.

There are several available models. Particularly useful in managing risk is the commonly used SWOT analysis of strengths, weaknesses, opportunities and threats. There are also more intuitive approaches, notably those which attempt to identify readiness for change, and the extent of commitment and support amongst those involved.

Transformational approaches to change, such as Total Quality Management and Business Process Re-engineering have a history in the NHS, but interventions at group or individual level are thought to be the way forward, particularly when clinician involvement is needed. Engaging people properly in the change process as teams and as individuals, rather than imposing the change upon them, influences the short and long term success of change programmes.

Individual attitudes to change are affected by how they perceive change affecting them, for example in terms of increased workload, loss of control or uncertainty. These perceptions can become reasons for resisting change. Change agents, generally managers, can reduce the risk of resistance to change by greater sensitivity to others' perceptions, or view of the risks to them, by ensuring support from influential members of the organisation, and by improving the quality of implementation.

The concept of the learning organisation is helpful to consider. Organisations often view themselves as learning organisations at times of significant change. For example, some newly created primary care groups and trusts (PCGs and PCTs) focused on developing themselves as learning organisations as a way of engaging the whole workforce in the change process. Successful PCTs have developed a culture which enhances opportunities for staff involvement and promotes learning from experience. This fosters strong innovative cultures, which are able to assess risks and learn from experience for the benefit of the wider healthcare community.

Project management 3.3

Project management provides a structure for organisational change irrespective of the level, nature or size of project. This approach can be used for any significant task that has an end objective. It is particularly important where major change (for example, implementation of the new consultant contract) takes place against a background of other day-to-day activities, and needs to be given the priority and resource to ensure success.

Key stages in project management are:

- Defining the purpose, objectives and deadlines.
- Identifying the resources needed.
- Assessing risks.
- Developing the project plan, milestones and key activities.
- Monitoring progress.
- Reviewing outcomes.

A project management approach should include the identification and assessment of risk, and the development of risk management strategies or contingency plans.

Drivers for change   3.4

The NHS employs over 1.3 million people, with a wide range of roles, training backgrounds, regulatory frameworks and accountability. This is the world's third largest workforce, after the Chinese red army and the Indian railways.[2] The NHS is also Europe's largest employer and is a complex organisation, with a great variety of cultures, working arrangements, customs and practice.

There is also a constant drive for change within the healthcare sector, whether management tier restructuring, service reconfiguration, or more simply, changes to the way people work. While there may be political drivers for change, for example, reduction in management tiers, costs, waiting list size or waiting time, in today's world of workforce pressures, the current NHS Plan (SEE KEY REFERENCES, APPENDIX 1) acknowledges that success may only be achieved by creating real changes in behaviour and work processes. Indeed, if we examine the NHS Plan and the modernisation agenda, increasingly, the need to do things differently becomes the main driver.

The NHS Plan   3.5

The NHS Plan is a ten-year programme of investment and reform published in 2000, to achieve a devolved service offering wider choice and greater diversity. Next steps[3] are increasing devolution to the frontline, strategic shifts to primary care, creation of the first Foundation hospitals, and different relationships between health and social services.

This programme of change will affect all healthcare organisations, either by mergers or reconfigurations. While the impact on individuals may vary, almost all will be affected by the human resource changes, notably pay modernisation and changes in job roles through the working differently programme.

People management – the impact of change   3.6

The NHS Human Resources (HR) strategy[4] is a vision for growing and developing the workforce to deliver faster and more accessible care based on patient choice. There are four key areas, which support the strategy:

- Pay and rewards.

- Learning and personal development.

- Regulation.

- Workforce planning.

Action in these areas has been identified as important contributors to successful change management, and the continuation of safe clinical practice.

Pay and rewards – Agenda for change   3.7

Agenda for change is a new pay system and three-year pay deal relevant to most NHS staff, excluding doctors, dentists and some senior managers. The new pay system is supported by a new job evaluation system and the Knowledge and Skills Framework (KSF) to provide a means of recognising the skills and knowledge required for particular jobs – aiming to make better links between training and development, career development and pay progression.

Agenda for change will provide harmonised terms and conditions for NHS workers and aims to address the issue of equal pay for work of equal value. Equal value claims over the past few years (for example those lodged by Speech and Language Therapists which progressed to the European Court of Justice) have exposed the NHS to risk. The new pay system aims to introduce a fairer system for determining basic pay by job weight.

Job weight will be assessed using a new job evaluation scheme, which measures 16 factors covering:

- The knowledge and skills required to do the job.
- The responsibility involved.
- The physical, mental or emotional effort.
- The extra demands imposed by the work environment.

Agenda for change is anticipated to be an extensive and lengthy change programme involving twelve early implementer sites before the new pay system starts to be rolled out across all health employers in 2004.

Getting pay and reward right can smooth the path to change. However there are risks to be managed with such an extensive change programme running parallel to others. These include the staff and management time required to evaluate jobs, distracting attention from other management tasks. Costs will be high, in terms of the three-year pay deal, job evaluation outcomes and training/implementation time. There will also be employee relations tensions if outcomes are not as expected, and possible legal claims.

Human resource specialists and other managers can learn from the current experience of implementing the new consultant contract. Important lessons are:

- Dedicating competent management resource for a high volume programme.
- Ensuring accurate financial and employment information.
- Establishing help lines to deal with queries in a consistent way.
- Setting up networks to monitor developments, promote good practice and avoid 'quick fixes'.

Properly implemented, *Agenda for change* is anticipated to be a key modernising lever for patient care. It will impact on almost everyone in today's health service.

Learning and personal development 3.8

Part of the lifelong learning strategy for the NHS, this programme aims to develop the skills and competences of all healthcare staff, including those who do not have professional qualifications, in partnership with social care, higher education and the newly launched NHS University.

Learning is important for organisational change as it boosts morale. Learning builds confidence and self esteem. People feel more fulfilled and see the opportunity to make a difference in the organisation.

Key features of the national programme include:

- New pre-registration programmes – in physiotherapy, occupational therapy, radiography, podiatry, speech and language therapy.

- Modernising medical careers – reform of the basic training grades and appraisal for all medical staff.

- Local pilots – nurse cadet and refugee doctor schemes.

This is a high profile national strategy, but there are local risks, which could compromise success, particularly if personal development plans are not rolled out to all staff, and appraisal is badly handled. Recent research from Aston University found a positive correlation between appraisal and organisational success, but also found that if appraisals are badly done, this has a negative effect. This reinforces the importance of management training in appraisal skills.[5]

Regulation 3.9

The NHS Plan includes reform of regulatory bodies and addresses cases of poor performance in order to restore public confidence following the highly publicised tragedies of the 1990's. Recent legislation has brought into effect new or reformed regulatory bodies:

- Nursing and Midwifery and Allied Health Professions Council.

- Council for the Regulation of Healthcare Professionals.

- Postgraduate Medical Education and Training Board.

- Reform of the General Medical Council.

- National Clinical Assessment Authority.

NHS employers will have to work with these new and reformed bodies to translate the benefits to frontline services, and adapt their own regulatory checking and referral processes. This particularly applies while the new organisations are in transition, and building up their own levels of competence. Not all services or functions will be immediately available, with a risk of lack of detailed advice for use locally.

Workforce planning   3.10

The new Strategic Health Authorities and Workforce Development Confederations have put together local delivery plans for the development of the healthcare workforce – part of the retention, workforce expansion and skill escalation agenda. However these organisations themselves are now to be integrated, resulting in a further change management programme running alongside the workforce planning agenda.

What are the risks of organisational change?   3.11

The sections above have aimed to outline the extent of the modernisation agenda at this point in time, and the implications for structural and process change. Some of the risks have already been identified, and these and others are reviewed further here.

Organisational health   3.12

Experience from industrial relations in the United Kingdom indicates that the impact of an announcement of organisational change is invariably perceived in terms of downsizing and rationalisation, with the possibility of redundancy, watching others leave, a loss of status or job satisfaction. Morale falls, and may undermine the productivity or other gains behind the change.

Risk factors[6] affecting morale and organisational health in general have been identified as including:

- Apparent unfairness over selection for redundancy.

- Survivors left unclear about what is expected of them.

- Lack of career development options.

- Alienation by cultural divides between merging organisations.

Practical solutions are around communications about the change, and support to survivors and leavers. Managers must be well informed and able to handle queries from staff, and deal with any problems within teams. It is important to monitor staff turnover, absence from work, customer service, productivity and performance, and other feedback as indicators of organisational health.

Poor organisational health impacts on performance and productivity, but decision makers often seem to play down the people and cultural issues in organisational change – in the early stages these are viewed as less important than dealing with negotiations over price, financial or legal structuring of the deal or contract.

Financial risks affecting people – pension liabilities, relocation and redundancy costs, as well as the costs of losing key people – are often not taken into account. The reason why retention, people costs and morale are neglected is because human resources (HR) is often left out of the loop[7] – left to pick up the pieces rather than influencing key decisions. Yet research on successful international mergers and acquisitions shows how early HR intervention can be key to integrating cultures successfully. In particular, human resource policy can mitigate some of the risks arising from the effect of the pace of change on individuals, and its impact on healthcare delivery.

Pace of change   3.13

Over half of the respondents to the recent Audit Commission report[8] on recruitment and retention in the public sector said that the number of change initiatives had been a deciding factor in their decision to leave their jobs. The report also highlights the extent of the pace of change, finding that a majority of those working in the health sector reported major organisational change in their workplace in the previous year. New initiatives were often seen as 'government initiatives' and viewed as an external imposition rather than a locally owned priority, or a continual cycle of change – seen as reinventing the wheel, with structures or solutions coming round again. This does not mean that people are opposed to change; rather that many perceive it as a distraction from 'what really matters' ie providing services to patients, and resulting in increased bureaucracy and paperwork.

The lessons from this research are clear, particularly around staff involvement and communications. Failure to 'sell' change as a contribution to service improvement, and the relevance of measurement and monitoring, will impact on morale and retention, with increased absenteeism and stress. There is a need for genuine local ownership, achieved by mainstreaming the change agenda and taking every opportunity to promote the rationale, involve staff at all levels, and celebrate success.

Role of pay and conditions   3.14

The Audit Commission Report also found a complex relationship between pay and motivation among public sector workers. While pay was cited as the biggest factor that could have enticed leavers to stay, few people in the public sector said that pay influenced their choice of job. For most it was the job itself, plus feeling valued and having the ability to make a difference, which mattered.

Public sector workers are also more likely to weigh up the whole package when deciding on whether to take a job, looking at hours of work, training, pension, annual leave, and whether the job itself is rewarding.

This is why the success of national initiatives like *Agenda for change* is crucial for the success of the health change agenda. People want a level of pay that accurately reflects their responsibilities, but this is only part of the overall reward package. Work life balance and personal development is just as important for public sector workers.

This is the rationale behind *Improving Working Lives*, a national programme requiring NHS organisations to introduce a wide range of policies and procedures that improve the working lives of their staff. These include initiatives on childcare, flexible retirement and flexible working, family friendly policies, valuing diversity and zero tolerance (bullying and harassment).

Employee relations   3.15

Workers in the public sector are more likely to belong to a union; 59% are members of a trade union compared to only 19% in the private sector. They are also more likely to be covered by a collective agreement. In NHS organisations, there are well-established recognition agreements, which provide for joint consultation with recognised trade unions.

The Government report[9] following consultation on the *European Information and Consultation Directive* (*EC Directive 2002/14/EC on a general framework of informing and consulting employees in the European Community*) acknowledges that effective employee dialogue can help staff feel more involved and valued by their employer, better aware of the business climate in which the organisation operates, and help them to be more responsive to, and better prepared for change. The consequences of a breakdown of employer-employee relations in a process of modernisation have been seen recently in the context of industrial disputes in the fire and postal services.

The *EC Directive on Information and Consultation* is to be phased in through UK legislation from 2005 depending upon the number of employees in the organisation. The Directive establishes a right to new minimum standards for workforce communication and involvement, including the right to be consulted on important decisions and to have access to information that could directly impact on working lives.

The detail of the impact for NHS organisations is unclear while the Government consults on options for implementation, and existing national and local mechanisms are likely to overlap with the new regulations. However, the new arrangements are predicted to expand the range of change issues which employees will have a right to be consulted on, and raise the profile of consultation with individuals who are not union members.

In anticipation of these new rights, good practice is to involve employees in change at the earliest opportunity, through the Joint Consultation Committee and consultation with any other staff organisations representing groups affected by change. Individuals should also be consulted, either by direct correspondence or open communication such as newsletters.

There is always the risk that disputes may arise during the change management process, and employers must ensure they have access to expert advice on collective dispute resolution and trade union rights.

Psychological contract 3.16

The psychological contract is a term used to describe a model of employment relations based on a notion of exchange – on a set of reciprocal obligations, promises and commitments between an individual or group of employees and their employer. The psychological contract is increasingly used as a way of exploring and understanding employment relations.[10] The state of the psychological contract amongst any group of workers or in an organisation is measured by looking at whether these implied promises, for example, on the part of the employer to introduce family friendly policies, and for the employee to respond with greater commitment, have been delivered.

Organisational change tends to be seen in terms of major restructuring. Yet in the public sector, there are a variety of types of change that can impact on the individual. These include reorganisation of work, new technology, changes in leadership and management style, cultural change, as well as outsourcing, mergers, take-overs and increased involvement of the private sector.

Change may be major or minor in its impact on individuals and on the state of the psychological contract. Major change is associated with a less friendly climate, and with lower levels of procedural fairness. This can be mitigated by action to improve organisational support and job security. If change is not seen as well handled, this will also increase negative attitudes to change.

However, on the positive side, change can also be associated with higher motivation and more opportunity to express views. Where change is to do with teams and the way people work with colleagues, individual responses can be particularly positive. A positive state of the psychological contract is also associated with an organisational climate that is perceived as friendly, fair, dynamic and less bureaucratic.

This indicates that the challenge for healthcare boards and managers is to focus on handling change effectively, which means dedicating greater resource and developing competence.

Legal framework 3.17

During organisational change, there are some employment rights, which assume significance. This section aims to summarise the law on transfer rights for individuals, and the emergence of the two-tier workforce, and the law on transfer of liabilities in healthcare organisations.

Transfer of Undertakings (TUPE)   3.18

The *Transfer of Undertakings (Protection of Employment) Regulations 1981 (SI 1981/1794)* (TUPE) aim to protect the rights of employees when their employment is transferred from one organisation to another. Within healthcare this can take place when trusts merge or new bodies are created as has happened recently with the Health Protection Agency (HPA). The TUPE regulations can also apply when only part of an undertaking is transferred.

The regulations are complex but broadly provide that wherever there is a transfer of an undertaking, the effect is that:

- The contracts of employment of the employees in the undertaking, or part of the undertaking, transfer to the new employer, as if they had always existed between the employee and new employer.

- The new employer must honour the existing terms and conditions of employment of the transferring employees, with the exception currently of pension entitlement.

- Any dismissal connected with the transfer will be automatically unfair, unless the dismissal is for an economic, technical or organisational reason (ETO reason). *Berriman v Delabole Slate Ltd [1985] ICR 546* established that an ETO reason includes changes to the numbers or functions of employees. Therefore redundancy will generally be an ETO reason where there is a reduction in the number of employees required to carry out work of a particular kind.

For healthcare organisations involved in outsourcing, mergers, reprovision of services or restructuring, the issue has always been to determine whether or not TUPE applies. Where the new provider already has employees able to do the new work, or there is pressure to downsize, there has often in the past been resistance from new employers to agreeing that TUPE will apply.

Understanding whether TUPE applies or not broadly involves answering a number of questions:

- Is the transfer area an undertaking?

  In deciding what an undertaking is, *Spijkers v Gebroeders Benedik Abbatoir CV (C24/85) [1986] ECR 1119; [1986] CMLR 296* has highlighted that the question to be asked is whether there is an identifiable economic entity to be transferred. Managers therefore have to look at the facts in each case.

- Is there a transfer?

  The key question is whether the entity retains its identity after transfer. Points to look for include:

  - Do tangible assets transfer e.g. buildings or equipment?

  - Do customers or clients transfer?

○   Are employees taken on by the new employer?

○   Do business contracts transfer?

○   How similar are the activities carried on after transfer?

Which employees will transfer? 3.19

People employed in the undertaking immediately before the transfer, will have the right of transfer. This includes both permanent and temporary staff, and those working under a contract of service.

The issue for health employers has usually been to determine which people are assigned to the transfer area. Difficulties always arise where part of an organisation is to be transferred, or where only part of an individual's job is in the transfer area. There are no specific rules on this. Current guidance is that if an employee is predominantly associated with that entity, they will probably transfer.

Individual cases are usually resolved as part of the consultation process, resulting in an agreed schedule of staff assigned to the transfer area on the day of transfer.

There is a wealth of case law on the application of TUPE, particularly regarding contracting – out, and the meaning of a transfer of an undertaking.[11] For the transferee (new organisation) there are also risks and liabilities which are outlined below.

Pensions 3.20

The right to membership of an occupational pension scheme does not currently transfer under the TUPE regulations. This is always a particular difficulty where individuals are being transferred out of the NHS to the private sector, and this contributes to resistance to the change. Guidance for the public sector[12] is that the new employer must offer transferring staff membership of a pension scheme which is 'broadly comparable' to the public sector scheme which they are leaving. Actuarial advice must be sought, generally from the Government Actuary's Department.

Redundancy 3.21

Redundancy benefits under the General Whitley Council agreement will also transfer as part of individual terms and conditions. This includes early retirement benefits on redundancy, which is a costly liability for new employers.

Statutory rights and liabilities 3.22

Liability between an employer and employee is also transferred, for example liability for personal injury arising out of accidents at work prior to transfer and any Employment Tribunal claims.

Collective agreements   3.23

Any recognition or collective agreement between the old employer and the transferring employees will also transfer and will apply unless the agreement is lawfully
ended. *Agenda for change* (NHS pay modernisation) is a collective agreement, and
it is therefore likely that individuals whose jobs would have been re-graded under
this before transfer, will argue that their new employer must comply.[13]

Terms and conditions   3.24

All contractual terms e.g. rights to salary, holiday and sick pay will also transfer. If
a change to terms and conditions occurs, case law has held the change may be
ineffective if the reason for the change is the transfer itself. This causes great difficulty if the new employer is seeking to harmonise terms and conditions with the
existing workforce, as there is no maximum period in law under which a dismissal
or change in terms and conditions may be said to be unconnected with the
transfer.

Consultation   3.25

Whenever there is a TUPE transfer, the transferor is required by the regulations
to give certain information to employee representatives. This includes information about any measures the employer envisages taking in relation to such
employees. A duty to consult with a view to reaching agreement also arises in
these circumstances. In the NHS, the duty to inform and consult is generally
incorporated in established organisational policies and procedures, which will
need to be reviewed for each organisational change.

Staff Transfers in the Public Sector – Statement of Practice   3.26

The Cabinet Office Statement of Practice issued in January 2000 aims to remove
some of the uncertainty over whether TUPE applies in various public sector situations, and facilitate modernisation, in particular, Public Private Partnerships
(PPP).

Policy in the statement is based on the following main principles:

- Contracting out exercises with the private sector and other public sector or
  voluntary organisations will generally be conducted on the basis that TUPE
  applies.

- This includes second and subsequent round contracts and where a function
  is brought back into the public sector.

- Where TUPE does not apply in strict legal terms the principles of TUPE
  should be followed to ensure individuals are not disadvantaged.

The statement of practice applies directly to the NHS, and clarifies the position particularly on transfers as a result of Public Private Partnerships, and second and subsequent transfers.

The two-tier workforce   3.27

One effect of TUPE, which follows the transfer of an undertaking, is the creation of a two-tier workforce.[14] The 'two-tier workforce' is the term used to describe an employment situation where staff performing the same role, in the same workplace, are employed on different terms and conditions. This situation exists in the NHS, as in other public sector organisations, as a result of outsourcing and organisational change. It impacts on patient care through the affect on morale, employee relations and staff retention.

This situation arises because:

● TUPE ensures it is difficult for the new employer to alter the terms and conditions of the transferred workforce.

● New (and existing) staff do not have this protection, and can therefore be employed on different employment terms.

This is a particular issue for public sector trade unions, who highlight that the UK is the only European member state which does not link public procurement to guaranteed labour standards. Trade union concerns centre on fears that the new employer will eventually harmonise pay and conditions to the detriment of former public sector employees. Generally this impacts on 'soft facilities management' – the semi- and non-skilled staff groups like cleaning staff.

Concerns about the two-tier workforce have been a barrier to change in the public sector. Initiatives to address this include the Retention of Employment model in the NHS, and the Best Value Review Code of Practice[15] in local government.

Currently the Retention of Employment model allows for a secondment arrangement for non-supervisory/managerial staff (domestics, porters, caterers, security, laundry and linen staff) in a Private Finance Initiative (PFI) situation. Secondees are regarded as employees of the NHS, but are managed on a day-to-day basis by the private sector PFI consortium. This enables staff to retain their NHS employment status and access to the NHS pension scheme. However there is a question over the long-term sustainability of the Retention of Employment model. External secondment arrangements are hard to manage, and further tiers to the workforce can emerge, for example managers, supervisors and 'hard facilities management' staff, such as estates staff, who often transfer on their own terms, and new starters.

In local government, the Best Value Review Code of Practice requires new joiners to be offered terms and conditions which are overall no less favourable than those of transferred employees. The Code aims to ensure that private sector involvement in the public sector is not at the expense of terms and conditions, and therefore not at risk of undermining service improvement. It is therefore a factor to be taken into account when local authority staff transfer under PPP schemes which also include NHS employees.

Private Finance Initiative (PFI)   3.28

A major change within the healthcare sector has been the introduction of the Private Finance Initiative in 1997. Partnerships between the public and private sectors are central to the achievement of the Government's modernisation programme.[16] Most major hospital projects, like schools, prisons, roads and computer systems, are now funded this way.

PFI is seen by Government as the most cost effective way to provide new hospitals and other public services without the need to increase the public sector borrowing requirement. It is further seen by Government as giving a much needed boost to the UK construction industry and as a way to introduce private sector expertise into the public sector.

Healthcare representative bodies have expressed concern about PFI funded projects, such as PFI funded hospitals leading to reduced bed numbers, pressures on staffing budgets, increased workloads and dilution of skill mix with the consequential impact upon patient care. Questions have also been raised about whether the PFI is an affordable long-term strategy for increasing capital investment in the NHS and is the best way to meet future healthcare demands.

The PFI is therefore an example of a major change initiative, imposed upon the NHS, and associated with less than whole-hearted commitment from all those working in the NHS. From the wider risk management perspective, this is not an ideal background to the effective introduction of major change. However, this is not to say that PFI funded projects in healthcare cannot be successful. Many such projects have now been completed and their success owes much to the energy, commitment and effective collaboration of those involved from both the healthcare and private sectors.

The National Audit Office (NAO) has published good practice guidance on successful partnerships in PFI projects.[17] The report is based upon a survey undertaken by the NAO into 121 PFI projects of which 44 were in the healthcare sector. Key points in the report relate to:

- The need for a partnership approach between the public and private sectors.
- Greater understanding of public and private sector strengths and business processes.
- An agreed and accurate contract.
- Appropriate allocation of risk.
- Inclusion of service quality statements in contractual conditions.

- Agreed mechanisms for dispute resolution.

- Change management procedures.

The need for an effective partnership between the private and public sectors cannot be over stressed. PFI partners need to recognise that they have a shared goal and different skills to bring to the achievement of that goal, whether in relation to a new hospital or a hospital ward. Whilst it is necessary for PFI partners to have a clear understanding of their respective roles up to project completion, it is equally necessary to achieve this once the project becomes operational.

Major PFI projects typically involve a private sector consortium, the precise make-up of which varies, but can involve bankers or other financiers, a construction company and facilities management specialists. It may therefore be necessary for healthcare staff to establish effective relationships with all or several members of the consortium. This adds to the complexity of developing a partnership approach and ultimately to the effective management of risk. In practice it is necessary to establish a number of groups or forums with appropriate representation from the PFI partners to assign responsibilities and check that agreed actions have been implemented.

Risk transfer is a characteristic of PFI contracts and involves the transfer of risk to the partner best placed to manage the risk. There is the potential for PFI partners to disagree about risk transfer; contractors may feel that too much risk has been transferred to them and healthcare partners may be too prescriptive in how the project is to be undertaken and in so doing retain responsibility for risk. This further underlines the need for effective communication between partners and agreement on respective roles and deployment of expertise.

Transfer of liabilities   3.29

When an NHS Trust is dissolved, either because of a transfer or reconfiguration of services, or Trust mergers, there are complex legal, financial and operational issues concerned with the transfer of liabilities.

A broad summary of the main legislation is in **TABLE 3.1**.

Table 3.1: Transfer of liabilities – main legislation

Legislation	Effect
The *National Health Service and Community Care Act 1990*	Provides for the Secretary of State to make an order to dissolve a trust and allows discretion on the transfer of property, rights and liabilities amended as below).
The *National Health Service Trusts (Consultation on Dissolution) Regulations 1991 (SI 1991/1347)*	Provides for the consultation required before an order is made

The *National Health Service Trusts (Consultation on Dissolution) Amendment Regulations 1992 (SI 1992/2905)*	Adds 'staff interests' to the consultation process
The *NHS (Residual Liabilities) Act 1996*	Sets out arrangements to deal with all outstanding liabilities if an NHS Trust, Health Authority or Special Health Authority ceases to exist. Ensures no liabilities remain untransferred, by removing Secretary of State discretion and replacing it with a duty to ensure all liabilities are transferred to other specified bodies, or to the Secretary of State.

The *NHS (Residual Liabilities) Act 1996* is considered of particular relevance in relation to the Private Finance Initiative as it removes any uncertainty for investors or contractors if there were to be a future reconfiguration of services.[18] Until this Act, legislation had left at the Secretary of State's discretion the future of any property, rights and liabilities if an NHS trust or other body were to be dissolved or abolished. Although there had been no cases where the Secretary of State had not exercised discretion to transfer liabilities, with the 1996 Act, there is now a duty to ensure that all liabilities are transferred to specified bodies or to the Secretary of State. At that time, there were over £1.5 billion worth of schemes seeking private finance in the NHS. Fifty-six schemes had been approved, with private sector capital commitments of more than £500 million. The new legislation was therefore important in reducing financial liabilities and promoting change.

The Department of Health checklist on transfer of liabilities covers:

- **Legal issues** – ensuring the establishment order contains the right details and is ready to be issued by the operational date of the new organisation.

- **Financial duties** – includes assigning a successor organisation to receive or repay brokerage.

- **Residual body** – addresses responsibility for claims and other legal liabilities, responsibility for the annual report and annual public meeting, and continuity of human resources input.

- **Charitable funds** – issues include Charities Commission liaison on registration and funds.

- **Funding issues** –includes assignment of income streams, allocation of corporate overheads and redundancy costs.

- **Expenditure** – the assignment of long-term contracts (maintenance, domestics, catering etc) and closure of bank accounts.

- **Transfer of fixed assets** – includes confirming current ownership and identifying future owners.

- **Current assets/liabilities** – issues include arrangements for the sale of current assets and the writing off of bad debts.

- **Other risks/liabilities** – for example, proper handover of fraud investigations, clinical negligence settlements, inventory lists, internal audit arrangements.

Involved organisations must make sure that there is a detailed project plan and overall co-ordination on progress and timescales.

Trust dissolution case study – Anglian Harbours NHS Trust 3.30

Anglian Harbours was a 'first wave' trust established in 1991 serving the eastern seaboard of Norfolk and Suffolk. The trust was dissolved in 1997 following a history of difficult relationships with the purchasers of its services. There were concerns about management costs, delivery of the trust's mental health services, medical staff cover, and training of junior doctors.

There were also internal disputes within the trust board. In one highly publicised incident in 1993, the chief executive resigned, and local trade union members picketed the trust headquarters.

The subsequent dissolution and transfer of services to neighbouring trusts was estimated to cost £3 million (excluding the change management costs for the new providers) and 63 staff lost their jobs through redundancy.

The establishment of NHS trusts under the *National Health Service and Community Care Act 1990* was a flagship change management programme, with the introduction of an NHS internal market, purchaser/provider split, and transfer of ownership and management to local service providers.

There was much pressure to move the trust programme forward. Anglian Harbours was one of the first trusts, and the business case and arrangements for the trust was probably not subjected to the same rigorous examination as was applied to subsequent rounds of trust applications. This has been a lesson learnt for the later creation of new organisations, for example Primary Care Trusts and Foundation Trusts, which have rigorous approval processes to ensure robustness and fitness for purpose.

The change process 3.31

The transfer of services from Anglian Harbours was achieved within a project management structure, in which a plan for dissolution was defined, accountability was apportioned and the timeframes and milestones determined. The need for strong communications to support the process was recognised at an early stage, with a regular news bulletin, staff road shows and open forums for staff at risk of redundancy. There were human resources policies introduced specifically to deal with the dissolution of the trust, covering:

- joint consultation arrangements;

- staff transfers; and

- avoidance of redundancy.

The consultation process produced few responses, raising doubts about how meaningful the consultation process was, given that those consulted were faced with a virtually irreversible situation. After consultation, the Secretary of State issued the *Anglian Harbours NHS Trust Dissolution Order 1997 (SI 1997/1987)* which dissolved the trust on 1 October 1997. One of the transferee trusts was appointed to act as the residual body to complete the dissolved trust's accounts and meet outstanding financial and other liabilities. A specific provision for this was made through the *Anglian Harbours NHS Trust Dissolution Order 1997.*

What aspects of the dissolution were well handled?   3.32

The report[19] on the dissolution concludes these were:

- the ability to maintain continuity of care during the transfer to new providers;

- managing the dissolution as a project;

- the effort put into communications and human resource management;

- the outplacement support available to at risk staff through independent providers; and

- the negotiation and transfer of around 1,000 staff to the new provider employers.

In addition, trade union representatives expressed appreciation at the time for the information sharing and strong human resource policy development.

What could have been done better?   3.33

The following points were identified:

- reconfiguration created particular uncertainty in one part of the trust, creating difficulties for the transfer of services and employee relations in the successor organisation;

- staff support in particular departments;

- public relations activity;

- problems with getting the information needed for the new providers, such as the different terms, conditions and policies applicable to transferred staff; and

- identifying resources for the change management process.

While important lessons were learnt, the ramifications for the successor organisations were significant in assuming new services and inheriting staff with a variety of employment terms and conditions, working practices and local culture.

Trust mergers   3.34

Between 1997 and 2002 there were 99 trust mergers in England, 14 of these in London. Mergers are driven generally by the need to make organisations more viable and better service providers – by pooling resources, mergers can provide an opportunity to improve the quality and range of services.

Research by the London School of Hygiene and Tropical Medicine[20] looked at the processes involved in and impact of mergers in the NHS. The study interviewed 96 trust board members, clinicians, service and senior managers, and compared management costs. It also examined the risks to service delivery and development, management structures, and staff recruitment, retention and morale.

The study identified a number of positive aspects of mergers, including:

- creation of a larger pool of professional staff;

- more influence with other public sector bodies;

- increased opportunities for staff training; and

- enhanced professional networks.

However, the research also identified a detrimental impact on clinical care delivery because of a loss of focus on services, with some planned developments delayed by at least 18 months. The tendency for one trust's management team to dominate over the other resulted in friction. There were no reported improvements in clinical or managerial recruitment and retention, and differences in culture were a barrier to integration. Conflicting priorities increased both the workload and stress of staff. Two years after mergers, target savings in management costs had also not been achieved.

To summarise, unless properly planned, resourced and managed, in the short term, mergers can cause considerable disruption to services, require greater management support, and take longer for a positive impact to be perceived. These lessons are important for risk avoidance in organisations undergoing restructuring, for example Primary Care Trusts taking on responsibility for general medical services.

Primary Care Groups and Trusts   3.35

A major feature of recent NHS organisational change has been the establishment of Primary Care Groups (PCGs), a total of 481 were created in 1999 and their later progression to Primary Care Trust (PCT) status. Initially operating as sub-committees of Health Authorities, as trusts they became responsible for their own budgets, the management and provision of community based services and the commissioning of hospital services for their local population.

The establishment of PCGs and PCTs was a major change from the NHS internal market of the 1990's. They were genuinely new organisations, and developing the vision of what they would look like, their roles and functions was time consuming. Information from leading PCGs about their activities and job roles was keenly sought by others and action to involve General Practitioners and their practice managers was important. Fostering a corporate spirit and identity with practititioners used to operating as independent entrepreneurs was, however, difficult.

It is significant that the three achievements most commonly cited by chief executives of PCGs in their first year[21] are:

- Building relationships with primary care professionals.

- Getting the board to work as a corporate group.

- Developing the organisation.

PCTs are still relatively small organisations and their ability to manage organisational development at the same time as improving services is related to their management capacity, particularly business and finance skills, and the availability of professional and support staff. Commentators believe this will continue until management constraints are resolved, and PCTs are able to pursue locally defined agendas.

Shared services and outsourcing   3.36

Shared service organisations are business units providing non – core functions (for example, finance, human resources, information management and technology) to a number of healthcare organisations.[22] Outside the health economy, many large multi-divisional companies have a history of working on shared services models, with cash releasing benefits, cost reduction and economies of scale, and using new e-business technologies.

In the NHS the National Shared Services Initiative was established in 1999, with the aim of exploring opportunities to improve the quality and value for money of non-clinical services. Early work focussed on governance arrangements, service level agreements and risk sharing arrangements. A main driver was the provision of support services to primary care organisations, to increase their management resource and capacity.

Anglia Support Partnership (ASP) is an example of a shared services organisation. Formed in April 2000 by a partnership of health organisations in Cambridgeshire and West Norfolk, ASP employs about 600 staff working across a variety of sites. Business activity includes the provision of facilities, finance, information management and technology, human resources and clinical governance services to eight NHS trusts, which between them employ over 5500 staff.

Shared services are essentially a form of outsourcing. The history of the NHS includes many examples of functions like laundry, catering and cleaning services shared by several local hospitals. Nationally, organisations such as NHS Estates and NHS Supplies have brought together scarce skills and purchasing power with the aim of improving quality and value for money.

However, the healthcare sector is generally nervous of outsourcing because of concern about the associated risk of whether outsourced functions can meet business requirements and those of the future market. Commercial organisations still tend to consider that keeping functions in-house carries a lower risk, but that may not be financially viable. Conversely in the public sector reduced commercial risk is generally perceived as less important when compared to the benefits from outsourcing or sharing services of improved business performance or service delivery. This is supported by evidence from the US that the correct outsourcing balance can reduce the drain on internal resources and impact on business performance.

However, many NHS Shared Services organisations are currently suffering from an increased perception of risk, particularly as primary care organisations grow in size and complexity. Many human resource functions are being drawn back in house as the workforce agenda priorities increase in importance.

Shifting the balance of power   3.37

The reorganisation of Health Authorities under the Shifting the Balance of Power (STBOP) exercise in 2002, involved moving staff and functions to new organisations, with many people assuming new roles, as part of the policy to shift resources and empower healthcare at the front line. The STBOP strategy illustrates how many of the lessons from previous restructurings are being taken on board.

For example, the principles of the STBOP change programme included:

- maintenance of service continuity while the change is managed;

- support for staff through the changes; and

- retention as far as possible of the skills, experience and commitment of existing staff.

Key early actions were:

- a project management, integrated approach;

- focus on cultural change and organisational development;

- leadership appointments and business plans; and

- communications with individuals.

Experience from the setting up of PCGs and trust mergers, where new roles created a mismatch with existing staff, resulted in clearing house systems being set up. This was to help displaced staff find employment in the wider healthcare sector or the Civil Service. Career counselling was provided, and partnership working established with trade unions. The emphasis in human resource policy and change processes was on transparency, fairness and equity.

In an effort to reduce the risk of redundancy, STBOP was notable[23] for the policy of a twelve-month period of guaranteed employment in order to find alternative employment for those posts declared redundant. The policy was intended to ensure adequate management resource during the change, and that no redundancies would be made during the twelve month period ending on 31 March 2003. It introduced an element of stability, but impacted on costs and morale while people were required to work in interim roles.

Foundation Trusts   3.38

The Government's aim[24] is that all NHS trusts will have reached a standard that will allow them to apply for NHS Foundation Trust status by 2008. NHS Foundation Trusts will be established in law as new legally independent organisations called public benefit corporations, with a duty to provide NHS services to patients, by the *Health and Social Care (Community Health and Standards) Act 2003.*

Foundation Trusts will be very different to other trusts in the healthcare sector; their legal base is different, and they will experience less Government control and enhanced local accountability. As such, the process of setting up Foundation Trusts involves a significant change agenda. For the first Foundation Trusts it means working towards outcomes of which there is little direct experience.

Governance arrangements, including the establishment of a Board of Governors, a Board of Directors, and Trust members are necessary.[25] Foundation Trusts also have the freedom to borrow to support their investment in service improvement.

If a Foundation Trust fails, it will be responsible for its liabilities and debts in the same way as a corporate plc. NHS Foundation Trusts will therefore need to ensure they have adequate indemnity arrangements to cover liabilities and debts and have effective risk management arrangements in place.

As far as liability of employees is concerned, according to common law, an employer is vicariously liable for the actions of employees when acting in that capacity. It is expected that NHS Foundation Trusts would also be vicariously liable for actions carried out by governors and non – executive directors in their capacity providing they are acting in good faith.

Care trusts 3.39

New organisations are coming into place designed to bring health and social care together. PCTs and local government social services functions are combining in parts of the country to offer new services, which in principle, means that groups like the elderly and disabled, will have their needs met in a more integrated way.[26]

The route to Care Trust status includes local consultation before a bid is put to the Department of Health, and a project management approach to implement the organisational and practical changes. Where Care Trusts have been established, it has often seemed a logical or natural progression for local services, due to a history of joint working.

However, at the end of 2003, there were only eight Care Trusts in place, and some concern about lack of uptake of this model. This reflects resistance to loss of local authority control of social services to Primary Care Trusts, and the electoral factor. Providing for local authorities to select the members who serve on care trusts has smoothed change, and some PCTs have elected co-opted members from the local acute and mental health trusts onto the board. It remains to be seen whether this model will succeed, but full integration, and a similar direction for children's trusts remains government direction.

The medical workforce change agenda

GMS contract 3.40

In 2003 the medical profession voted to accept a new General Medical Services (GMS) contract. The contract is far more than a method for payment to General Practitioners (GPs). Rather, it is viewed as a powerful tool for modernising primary care services and creating innovative change, in terms of workforce, infrastructure, commissioning services and information management and technology. The main drivers behind the new contract are the national shortage of GPs and the need for the primary care workforce to meet the demands of the modern NHS.[27]

Key changes include:

* Rewards to practices will in future be structured to benefit those offering higher quality care. This will include a global sum to cover running costs, quality payments to reward standards, and enhanced service payments for practices that expand the range of services they provide.

- Improvements to GPs working lives to improve recruitment, retention and morale, such as access to childcare provisions, parental, maternity and paternity leave, and sabbatical leave.

- A new career structure for GPs, including skills development and specialist roles, greater employment of salaried GPs and protected time for skill development.

- A wider range of services available to patients in the community, with the expectation that practice nurses will become specialist providers of front-line services to patients.

- PCTs will assume full responsibility for out of hours' services, as GPs will no longer be required to provide this cover. PCTs will need to ensure 24-hour care is available for all patients, is delivered to quality standards, and that integrated emergency care services are developed.

This is an extensive change agenda with real risks to continuity of patient care if, for example, satisfactory alternative out of hours and emergency services are not negotiated by PCTs; information technology systems are not adequate, or recruitment and retention of GPs and nurses does not improve significantly. There are concerns about consistency in the new arrangements, and capacity in PCTs and practices to deliver the change.

A model structure plan has been developed to help PCTs deliver on implementation of the new contract. Key stages include:

- Developing a consultation plan.

- Identifying dedicated management arrangements.

- Appointing a steering group.

- Using basic project management tools to map out a work programme.

- Devising a communications strategy.

- Identifying and involving other stakeholders with a claim, concern, risk or investment in the delivery of the new contract. This is particularly important for delivery of the GMS contract, where changes in emergency or specialist services provision will impact on nearby acute trusts, ambulance and paramedic services, NHS Direct and current out of hours' medical services.

- Arrangements for sharing learning and good practice, through networks of practices, nurse practitioners and human resource specialists.

Unless these arrangements are in place, there is a significant risk that capacity and resource at strategic level will not be available to ensure success.

The new consultant contract 3.41

NHS consultants working in hospital, community and public health services are excluded from *Agenda for change* but will be affected by the new consultant contract, which will impact on pay and the way in which senior doctors will work in the future.

The new contract is being introduced following past resistance from the medical profession, including at one time the threat of industrial action if the contract was imposed. In June 2002 the DoH and British Medical Association developed a framework document, but the medical profession rejected the proposals following a ballot in October. It took until the following year before new proposals were agreed in the Heads of Agreement document of July 2003 (SEE USEFUL WEBSITES BELOW). Consultants were encouraged to give a formal commitment to move onto the new contract by invitation and estimates of individual pay calculations. A second ballot in October 2003 resulted in a 60.7% yes vote.

The pay ramifications of the new contract are significant – up to a 24% pay increase for individual doctors, at an estimated cost of over £100 million in the first year for England trusts. Other costs, for example, salary backdating, extra programmed activities, reduction in the session length for out of hours work and phasing in of pay for maximum part-time consultants, are difficult to quantify. There are other non-pay ramifications, particularly the impact of agreed job plans and the new private practice code on service delivery (SEE USEFUL WEBSITES BELOW), making it difficult to currently judge if the contract will deliver on productivity for all specialties.

It is expected that the contract will affect the roles and responsibilities of other healthcare workers as working practices and consultants' hours of work change as a result. This impact will increase with the implementation of the *European Working Time Directive* (*Council Directive No 93/104/EC of 23 November 1993 concerning certain aspects of the organisation of working time*) on junior doctors' working hours, examined in the next section.

Changes in junior doctors' hours   3.42

Junior doctors, or doctors in training, currently provide a major input to frontline hospital service delivery, working long hours over a variety of night and day shifts and on-call cover. This situation, long of concern on risk management grounds, can no longer continue. Junior doctors' working hours have been limited by their contract to no more than 58 hours actual work on average per week since August 2003. From 1 August 2004 their exclusion from the 48 weekly working hours limit under the *European Working Time Directive* will be removed, and from that date a 58 hour limit will apply.

In addition, a recent judgement in the European Court of Justice,[28] known as the Spanish Doctors case (*Sindicato de Medicos de Assistancia Publica (Simap) and Conselleria de Sanidad y Consumo de la Generalidad Valenciana Case C-303/98*), has determined that all on-call time will be working time if a worker is required to be on-call at their place of work. This includes when the worker is sleeping, and has implications therefore for the working hours of all healthcare roles, such as sleep-in shifts by night staff in community homes.

This judgment has been confirmed by a further case (*Landehauptstadt Kiel and Norbert Jaeger Case C-151/02*), which in addition held that periods of compensatory rest for time worked in what would otherwise be rest time must immediately follow the period of work to which they relate.

These judgments increase the difficulty of achieving the working time limits for junior doctors, with the solutions already constrained because of shift structures, workload pressures and skill shortages .

There are risks to NHS employers if they fail to implement working time limits for junior doctors and risks if they do. Risks of non-compliance with legal requirements are unsafe working practices by tired doctors and the resulting clinical negligence claims are all possible outcomes. There is also a risk of proceedings by individuals through Employment Tribunals.

There are further risks if implementation of the change is badly managed. This could lead to a reduced quality and quantity of patient care, low morale and further pressure on training delivery because of restrictions when education can be delivered. Other staff may also risk exceeding the working time limits in order to ensure junior doctors are compliant.

There is no alternative to service reconfiguration in order to avoid associated risks, but effective management is necessary. The changes to be implemented will have far reaching consequences including the affect on local working patterns. These include:

- Implementing *Hospital at Night*, a competency-based model for teams working at night – this aims to identify the actual skill base required in individual hospitals at night based on healthcare risk, and ensure cover is provided by a the correct mix of clinical and non-clinical roles.

- Cover by non-medical practitioners and new types of healthcare worker.

- Cross cover for on-call between specialties and sites.

- Collapsing tiers of cover so that emergency care is provided by senior rather than junior staff.

- Greater use of multi-disciplinary teams.

These changes can be seen as part of the NHS *Changing Workforce Programme*, which is leading on the development and wider promotion of new roles as part of the modernisation agenda.

Summary   3.43

This chapter has aimed to analyse the extensive change management agenda currently in place to underpin modernisation of service delivery. This agenda includes fundamental changes to staff roles, working practices, reward and development, against a background of structural change and the shift of resources to frontline healthcare in primary and acute sectors. While this is happening, services to patients must continue to be both provided and developed, and national targets achieved.

If change programmes do not fully succeed, there is always the risk that the benefits in terms of service improvement will not be realised. There are also other human resources risks (impact on morale, retention, employee relations) with a wider impact if people are not engaged in the change programme.

Key actions to underpin organisational change and manage the risks
3.44

- Develop the corporate strategy, based on the business environment, identifying key stakeholders and change partners.

- Include in this process a robust, influential human resources policy.

- Implement a project management approach which includes risk assessment.

- Involve affected individuals in the process of change.

- Focus on communication and consultation.

- Put in place the right financial and management resource.

- Consider the people risks – especially stress, morale, motivation and retention.

Following these basic steps will contribute to effective management of change programmes, identification of risks and development of a robust strategy and action plan.

References

1 NCCSDO (May 2001) *Managing change in the NHS, organisational change, a review for healthcare managers, professionals and researchers*, London School of Hygiene and Tropical Medicine
2 'Smooth operation' (2003) People Management, 23 October.
3 HMSO (2002) *Delivering the NHS Plan.*
4 Department of Health (2003) *Delivering the HR in the NHS Plan 2003.*
5 NHS Magazine, (June 2003) 'Pride and progress'.
6 'Employee morale during downsizing' (1995) *IES Report*, 291.
7 CIPD (2003) *International mergers and acquisitions – a guide.*
8 *Recruitment and retention*, (2002) Audit Commission.
9 DTi (2003) *Information and Consultation Directive, Consultation: High Performance Workplaces: Informing and consulting employees.*
10 Guest DE and Conway N (2001) *Public and Private Sector Perspectives on the Psychological contract*, CIPD.
11 Hammonds Suddards Edge (2000) *Transfer of Undertakings*, CIPD.
12 Cabinet Office (2000) *Staff Transfers in the Public Sector, Statement of Practice.*
13 'Movers and shapers', (2003) *Health Services Journal*, 6 November.
14 Anderson R (2003) *The Two-tier Workforce*, New Health Network.

15   News Release, Office of the Deputy Prime Minister, 13 February 2003.
16   HM Treasury (2000) *Public Private Partnerships. The Government's Approach*, HMSO.
17   National Audit Office (2001) *Managing the relationship to secure successful partnership in PFI projects. Report by the Comptroller and Auditor General*, HC 375 Session 2001–2002: 29 November 2001.
18   Circular FDL (96) 30, NHS (Residual Liabilities) Act 1996, NHS Executive, June 1996.
19   Barrick A and Balcombe P (1998) *Anglian Harbours – the first NHS trust dissolution*, NHS.
20   Fulop N and others (2002) 'Process and impact of mergers of NHS Trusts: multicentre case study and management cost analysis', *BMJ*, 3 August.
21   Wilkin D, Gillam S, Smith K (2001) 'Tackling organisational change in the new NHS', *BMJ*, 16 June.
22   Shared Services, Management briefing, National Electronic Library for Health, April 2003.
23   'Reorganisation and redundancy payments' (2003) *Employment Law Register*, NHSP
24   Department of Health (2002) *A guide to NHS Foundation Trusts.*
25   *NHS Foundation Trusts, a guide to developing governance arrangements*, Department of Health, September 2003.
26   'Small but perfectly formed' (2003) *Health Service Journal*, 16 October.
27   NATPACT (2003) *The new GMS contract: moving to implementation.*
28   'Working Time Directive – status of periods of inactivity while on call', *IDS Brief*, November 2003.

Further information

Professor Sue Arrowsmith (Editor) (2001) *Public Private Partnerships & PFI*, Sweet & Maxwell

Useful websites

1   **The Private Finance Initiative (PFI):**

HM Treasury: www.hm-treasury.gov.uk

Office of Government Commerce: www.ogc.gov.uk

Department of Health: www.doh.gov.uk/pfi

National Audit Office: www.nao.gov.uk

2   **Checklist for the transfer of liabilities:**

http://www.info.doh.gov.uk

3   **Human resource framework: shifting the balance of power:**

http://www.doh.gov.uk

4   **Agenda for change:**

http://www.doh.gov.uk

5   **Improving working life:**

The GMS contract

Junior doctors hours

6   **Anglia Support Partnership:**

http://www.asp.nhs.uk

7   **The consultant contract:**

http://www.modern.nhs.uk/consultants

Chapter 4
Incidents: Recording, Analysis and Investigation

This chapter covers:

- Defining incidents.

- Methods for reporting incidents.

- Categorising incidents.

- Analysing data.

- Learning lessons from incidents.

- National Patient Safety Agency (NPSA) requirements.

Introduction   4.1

Much has been written on procedures for the identification, reporting and management of incidents or adverse events, but little on the critical evaluation of the effectiveness of incident recording as a risk management process. Many readers familiar with incident recording will have experienced frustration with the associated bureaucracy, and the inability to learn lessons from the incidents that have arisen and prevent their recurrence.

Some of this may be due to the reluctance of clinicians and managers to take incident data and analyse it to the extent that it yields valuable management information. One limiting factor is the quality and validity of data available to practitioners that provides the confidence in using it to base decisions on. Another complicating factor is the difficulty of differentiating truly high-risk incidents from the vast number of incidents that may be reported in a complex healthcare setting.

This chapter discusses the importance of and the principles of incident reporting, analysis and investigation. It discusses how it can be applied in a healthcare setting, its role as part of an internal risk management programme, its association with the national programme for patient safety and lastly, its value in terms of changing the culture of an organisation. This should enable readers to:

- develop incident definitions;

- understand why incident recording is an important component of any risk management strategy;

- develop an incident reporting programme that covers the recording, analysis and evaluation of data and links in with the national programme for reporting; and

- utilise incident information to influence change in an organisation and learn lessons and effect change.

This chapter focuses on the wide range of incidents that may occur in the healthcare sector, so that a better understanding of what information needs to be collected to inform change in an organisation can be gained.

What is an incident? 4.2

Standard dictionary definitions for the word 'incident' define it as a definite or distinct occurrence, or an event. In this context and for the ease of the reader, incident and event are used interchangeably throughout this chapter. A good working definition, that has been used successfully in NHS organisations is:

> 'any unexpected event that has an actual or potential detrimental effect on a patient, employee, member of the public or indeed the assets of an organisation.'

It is not unusual in healthcare for the recording of clinical events to be separate from non-clinical events. However non-clinical events may have a direct impact on a patient or related to a patient procedure. Sometimes this distinction is unhelpful, and can lead to energy being misdirected at how to record an incident, rather than learning lessons from the incident.

Accident or incident? 4.3

A distinction can be made between accident and incident. The reason behind this is to encourage a culture of reporting incidents where no harm may have occurred as opposed to only reporting those 'accidents' where harm has occurred. Accident refers to an event where there has been some damage, for example to individual(s) or to property.

DoH terminology 4.4

The Department of Health (DoH) has restated the importance of patient safety and crucially the importance of staff involvement and engagement in the process. The DoH has defined 'adverse healthcare events' (AHCE) and a 'healthcare near-miss' (HCNM). These were defined as follows and on p35 of *Building a Safer NHS for Patients*[1]:

- An adverse healthcare event is an event or omission arising during clinical care and causing physical or psychological injury to a patient.

- A healthcare near-miss is a situation in which an event or omission, or a sequence of events or omissions, arising during clinical care fails to develop further, whether or not as a result of compensating action, thus preventing injury to a patient.

The definition was further expanded in *Doing Less Harm*[2] where an adverse patient incident was defined as 'any event or circumstance arising during NHS care that could have or did lead to unintended or unexpected harm, loss or damage'.

More recently the DoH's National Patient Safety Agency (NPSA), established as a Special Health Authority, to improve the quality of care through the reporting, analysis and learning from incidents, has published its *Seven Steps to patient safety – a guide for NHS Staff*. The document encourages a common language for patient safety, which will be used in this chapter. These are direct quotes from the guidance.

'**Patient safety:** the process by which an organisation makes patient care safer. This should involve:

- risk assessment

- the identification and management of patient-related risks

- the reporting and analysis of incidents

- the capacity to learn from and follow-up on incidents

- implement solutions to minimise the risk of them recurring.

Patient safety incident: any unintended or unexpected incident which could have or did lead to harm for one or more patients receiving NHS funded healthcare. This is also referred to as an adverse event/incident or clinical error, and includes near misses.'

The NPSA definitions are consistent with the definition mentioned earlier in the chapter, but it is focused on patients who receive NHS funded care. Incidents, for the purposes of this chapter, will embrace the wider community including patients.

Strategic Health Authorities, as part of their performance management role in clinical governance, have tended to adopt different terminology, some using serious adverse events (SAE) and others, serious untoward incidents (SUI). Irrespective of the terminology used, being able to define and then classify an incident is important if this information is to be used to assess and manage risk. Near-miss incidents are extremely important to capture as they tell the story of what might have happened had the circumstances been different. The three-incident rule is a good one to go by – if a minor incident or near-miss has occurred three times, there will be a likelihood that the fourth event will be of a serious nature, although, in reality, a more serious outcome could happen at any time.

Why do people fail to report? 4.5

The difficulty with incident reporting appears to be in the process itself and how incident reporting systems are used. Incidents are reported every day in a variety of ways – the accident seen on the road and the subsequent phone call to the police, the leak in the washing machine, the scorched shirt during ironing or the present broken after a child's birthday party. We think nothing about telling others about these events. So why is it any different when we are in the work environment? Why is it that reporting of incidents, however insignificant, becomes something so difficult to do? It might be the fear of 'big brother', in other words people's perception that the 'organisation' is watching and therefore should not know too much about what goes on. This might preserve autonomy from those in authority, in order to maintain some sense of control in the workplace. Fortunately this type of thinking is not as prevalent in the NHS when risk management was first introduced in the early 1990's. Change has resulted from clinicians taking the lead to improve patient safety, greater patient empowerment and increased public awareness of clinical errors.

However, what of incidents that must be reported because there is a legal requirement to do so? The *Reporting of Injuries, Diseases and Dangerous Occurrences Regulations 1995 (SI 1995/3163) (RIDDOR)* requires the reporting of certain categories of incidents. Yet time and time again it can be shown that despite legal requirements, individuals and organisations continue to fail to report. This is often due to ignorance or a lack of understanding rather than malicious intent. Incident reporting is not seen as necessarily important or core to the business, when in fact it most certainly is.

Methods of reporting 4.6

There are many sources of guidance on how to report incidents – the use of forms, confidential telephone lines, in person, with or without a witness, by facsimile or through electronic databases. Then there is the question about which systems are preferable; for example, if a written form is to be used, what design is required to capture relevant incident information? The question of what is relevant information arises – or, in other words, what is the necessary data set required? There is also the question of who should see the form once completed and who is responsible for taking any action following the incident.

The National Patient Safety Agency has developed a standardised dataset and reporting forms that will be used to gather patient safety incident information. It will be rolled out during 2004 and will greatly improve the type and quality of data acquired and reported to optimise learning in the NHS. NHS organisations will continue to use their own incident reporting systems and will be able to participate in the national system. The following sections provide practical guidance for those wishing to adopt or revise a system, which as time progresses, should follow the national approach.

Designing incident forms   **4.7**

Opinions vary on the fields to include in incident reporting systems. With forms, for example, some prefer free text, but others wish to use tick-boxes or checklists. Opinions differ about whether there should be one form for all incidents or separate forms for clinical and non-clinical events and even separate forms within these subdivisions. It has been known, for instance to have a form for clinical incidents, another for accidents, another for violence and another for drug errors. A system that is complex from the outset will struggle because of the demands it will make on those who have to use it. It is unlikely that with a number of different reporting systems, full reporting will take place.

Those that have had experience of designing incident forms, will be familiar with the difficulties that arise during what appears to be a pretty straightforward process. Discussions can become very emotive and highly charged, especially concerning where organisational logos will appear – everyone becomes a graphic designer when incident forms are being developed! To avoid this, here are some key points to remember when setting up an incident reporting system for the first time or alternatively, when a system is being reviewed.

Developing an incident reporting system

Research existing systems   **4.8**

Before beginning the process, find out what is being done in the healthcare field on incident reporting. Gather information from healthcare organisations, for example, a large teaching hospital, district general hospital, primary care trust and family health practitioner services such as general practice or dentistry.

Explore what other industries have done. High-risk sectors, such as air and rail transport offer a lot when it comes to designing a process used by thousands of employees. Not only should the research look at what systems they are using, but also what their future plans are for reporting, analysis and improvement of the system. It is useful to consider the many incident reporting systems currently available as software packages. Most of these have not, however, been developed specifically for use in healthcare and one should use caution if moving to an untried system. The introduction of an integrated patient record may also have an impact on the type of incident reporting system installed as there may be a need to integrate the systems to reduce duplication of information.

Set the research in context   **4.9**

Information should be considered and set in the context of the organisation's work. For example, if the organisation is well advanced with computer hardware and software and has competent users, an electronic system for incident reporting is worth exploring. If not, then using a paper reporting system to begin with supported by a method of collating the data, normally through a database system, is preferable. Put a plan in place to move to electronic reporting in future, which will be sooner than you think. Always have a contingency plan particularly if reliant solely on electronic reporting (e.g. effective back-up systems).

Explore alternative systems   4.10

Other methods should also be explored, for example, the use of telephone reporting and confidential or anonymous ways of reporting events, especially critical ones. Auditing medical records is a good way of retrospectively identifying incidents and can be used as part of a peer review or appraisal process. This information should be added to the research information already gathered, critiqued and an analysis done on the research to date. The aim of this is to be as knowledgeable prior to embarking on a project to set up both internal and external incident reporting.

External incident reporting   4.11

External incident reporting will be required for example by RIDDOR. Strategic health authorities will want serious events reported, NHS trust boards will wish to publicise their performance on clinical safety and the DoH, through the National Patient Safety Agency, will have reporting requirements.

Involve staff and keep it simple   4.12

When a reporting system is about to be devised, staff should be involved. There is nothing more frustrating than to be involved at length in the development and introduction of a complex system and then find it is seen as an imposition by management and therefore part of some political, externally influenced ideology. This is a view that has been expressed over a number of years by clinicians and must be avoided if the aim is to improve patient and staff safety.

Healthcare professionals spend a considerable proportion of their day documenting information, so any increase in their workload through the introduction of another form must be done with care. Clinicians will have an opinion about what methods should be used. Their ownership of the process and involvement, particularly of doctors, will ensure the success of any incident reporting process.

Clinical staff are focused on what goes on in their environment and want any system that is introduced to be one that will support them, not distract them from their duties, where possible. This has to be a critical factor when considering the introduction of a reporting system – keeping the system simple, but with maximum effectiveness, is a good principle to abide by.

Communicate   **4.13**

Make sure that everyone, as far as possible, is aware that research into and development of an incident reporting system is taking place, why it is being developed and what their role in it will be.

- Tell staff who is being consulted and seek volunteers throughout the process.

- Use tried and tested communication methods such as newsletters, team briefings and email.

- Make sure there is a contact person in case there are questions.

- Give an indication of when the system will be introduced.

- Conclude with what training and education will be available to staff in order that the system is successful.

Putting policy and ideas into practice   **4.14**

Incident reporting is not a means to an end, but a tool that can be used to reduce risk and improve working practices. To let it become an industry is to lessen the importance of incidents and how they can influence and change the behaviour of individuals or an organisation itself.

The purpose of reporting is to learn the lessons of past mistakes and change working practice so that further incidents are avoided. Changing the culture of the organisation so that incidents are seen as a positive indicator of performance as opposed to a negative one is the objective to achieve. In **CHAPTER 2**, the organisation, the environment and the people involved were described as key to having an effective risk management strategy (see **FIGURE 2.3**). These three factors will be used as the basis to show how incident reports and improvements in risk and quality are linked.

Demonstrating how incidents work within the scope of risk management is best shown using the example of a medication or drug error that occurs in hospital.

Case study: medication error

Setting the scene   **4.15**

Patient B has been given medication prescribed for another patient, patient A, who is located in the same bay (see **FIGURE 4.1**).

Figure 4.1: Ward Layout for four patients

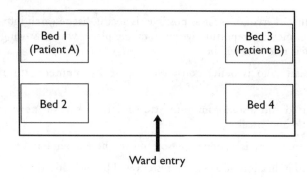

Patient A is located in Bed 1. Patient B is located in Bed 3. Due to staff shortages, a bank nurse is brought in to work the late shift. There is a policy in the hospital that any bank nurse has to be supervised in the checking of any medications, but if they have the appropriate experience, they can administer as part of a team.

At the nursing station there is a whiteboard with each bed number (there are 28 beds in all). Beside each bed number on the whiteboard is the patient's name and their assigned consultant.

All 28 beds are full with medical patients, and the average patient age is over 65. Some of the patients are very ill and therefore highly dependent on nursing care. On this particular shift, the bank nurse is assigned a number of bays with a particularly highly dependent caseload. There are two other qualified nurses on duty and one healthcare assistant.

What goes wrong? 4.16

Medications are checked following procedure and the bank nurse administers medication to patients in the first bay, numbered beds 1–4. The nurse checks the whiteboard for Patient A and the patient's location, satisfied that Patient A is in Bed 1. The nurse then proceeds with the medication to the bay, enters it and moves to Bed 3 rather than Bed 1 thinking that Bed 1 is on the right rather than the left.

The nurse approaches the bedside, asks the patient in Bed 3 if Patient A. The patient nods affirmatively and is given medication. The nurse, having checked that no other patients in the bay are due for medication, leaves the bay and documents the administration on Patient A's chart.

Patient B calls out sometime later and the healthcare assistant nearby attends the patient. Patient B asks why medication was given when the patient was sure their medication had finished. The healthcare assistant speaks to the bank nurse and then, through their conversation, it becomes evident that the medication given was not prescribed and, in fact, was given to the wrong patient.

Establishing the mistake   4.17

The nurse notifies the senior nurse on the ward and as they retrace the steps up to giving the medication, it becomes apparent that two fundamental errors were made. These were:

- The nurse made an assumption about the arrangement of the beds, believing that Bed 1 was located in the upper right hand corner of the bay, when in fact Bed 1 was in the upper left hand corner of the bay.

- The nurse asked the patient their name, and they appeared to respond in the affirmative. What the nurse did not do was actually check the patient's wrist identification band to confirm identity.

This second action compounded the initial error. The incident can be broken down and examined as to what may have gone wrong and how it could be prevented again. In this way, reporting and analysing an incident can be productive and used as an educational tool. In addition it can also lead to changes that may prevent the incident from occurring again and underlies the importance of root cause analysis, discussed in **CHAPTER 5** and one that will be promulgated via the National Patient Safety Agency.

Analysing the incident

The people   4.18

Those directly affected in the medication error incident are: the patient who received medication in error, the patient who did not receive their medication, the bank nurse and the senior nurse. The doctor was notified and observations were taken to make sure the patient did not suffer any ill effects. The error was recorded in the patient's medical record.

The nurse, as expected, was very upset and wary of proceeding with administration of any other medications on the ward. As a result, the senior nurse decided to supervise any further administrations. This caused some delay for the other patients as an unanticipated risk had now been introduced into the system (see **2.14** – Interdependency of risk).

The environment   4.19

From the case study described, the ward was busy and the bank nurse had a high case load of highly dependent patients. By investigating the incident, a number of issues were identified:

- The whiteboard with the bed numbers and patient names was not supported by an illustration of the bay layouts.

- The beds were not numbered.

- The bank nurse, who normally works on another ward was unfamiliar with this particular ward.

- Due to dependency of the patients and the ward being busy, the bank nurse was not given any instruction as to the layout of the ward before starting the shift.

- The nurse did not check the patient identification band to confirm the patient's identity.

- The nurse relied on the patient to confirm their own identity.

The organisation   4.20

Organisational risks, discussed in **CHAPTER 2**, include issues such as policy and procedures, and human resources – which would include recruitment and retention strategies, education and clinical supervision.

During the incident review, a number of findings about the organisation were exposed:

- Because of recruitment and retention issues, staffing was below the required level for the number and dependency of patients admitted. Therefore the ward manager relied on bank nurses (those employed within the hospital, but who are willing to work extra shifts) and/or agency nurses (those employed by another organisation that are contracted to work on hospital wards as and when required).

- There were no procedures in place to make sure that bank or agency staff working on the ward were given an induction of the ward.

- There were no procedures in place covering clinical supervision and the administration of medication. Instead it was up to the discretion of the senior nurse on duty to decide whether the bank nurse could administer medication.

The incident is a good learning tool for improving practice and the application of procedures. It is important to use the incident as a learning tool rather than seeking to allocate blame for the error itself.

Determining the level of risk   4.21

Considering the incident described, it would be easy to immediately classify it as serious or significant, but was it? This is where the subjectivity of assessing risk comes into play.

Had the patient been given a morphine-based medication that had the effect of lowering the respiration rate, the incident would be considered as serious. If the patient had been given a standard antibiotic with nil effect, then the incident could be graded as insignificant or of low risk. But what if the patient had been allergic to the antibiotic? The outcome could have been very significant, with the patient having an allergic reaction, or in the worst case scenario, dying. This illustrates why it is so important to prevent incidents such as medication errors arising, as the eventual outcome could be left to chance.

By considering different potential outcomes from the incident, through for example root cause analysis, it can be used as a learning tool to see how one error can multiply in magnitude. Using incidents in this way allows risk management to be a tangible, positive influence in making changes within an organisation without fear of retribution from others. Making incident reporting and learning a positive experience will make it a very effective tool in reducing risks within the organisation.

Recording and reviewing data 4.22

Incident reporting can be a force for good, but is not always seen as that, as organisational culture plays a key role in how incidents are dealt with. In the example, if blame had been apportioned for the incident and a warning issued to the bank nurse, the outcome might have been entirely different. This type of approach discourages an open culture which encourages and facilitates the reporting of incidents. A balance will need to struck between using the learning to promote patient safety set against cases where a practitioner has breached their duty of care or standards of competencies, which would require intervention through management (e.g. instituting clinical supervision).

Recording data 4.23

How should incident data be recorded if it is to be meaningful and of use to the organisation? The starting point will be to identify the minimum data set required for data collection.

Minimum data set 4.24

A minimum data set should be based on the principles of who, what, where, when, how and why the event or near-miss occurred.

- **Who or what was involved?** – identification of the person or persons affected or equipment or facilities involved.

- **What happened?** – a description of the incident itself based on fact, not opinion.

- **Where did it happen?** – the location of the incident and the clinical speciality involved.

- **When did it happen?** – time and date of the incident.

- **How did it happen?** – an explanation of how the event may have occurred based on an analysis of the event.

- **Why did it occur?** – this will take the analysis a step further to look at what the underlying or root cause might be and what factors may have contributed to the incident.

Other information that should be included in the data set is any action taken to deal with the situation and what level of risk associated with the incident. Incident reports should identify who reported the incident and when it was reported.

When to report data   4.25

Staff should be encouraged, if not instructed, as part of a policy and procedure on reporting, to report as soon as the event unfolds or is known about. This will allow those involved to discuss the incident with a clear sense of what happened, making it easier to understand and evaluate the incident. It will also provide a named person if further information is required, an important point if an investigation is required at a later date.

Form layout   4.26

The design of the form is important if an incident reporting programme is to be successful as part of a risk management and wider clinical governance strategy. A sample incident form is shown in **FIGURE 4.2** of how information can be recorded using a simple layout. This is a working example used in acute and primary care (with some slight alterations), developed on the premise that it needs to be simple and easy to complete yet capture the maximum amount of data possible. It is supported by a software system that allows meaningful statistics to be obtained with minimal effort.

Figure 4.2: Sample incident form

Date:	Time:	Location and speciality/department:
Name:		If Employee: Full time or part time? Hours worked Absent for > 3 days? Yes/No
Diagnosis (for patients): Type of injury sustained:		Consultant:
Describe what happened stating only fact, not opinion: Reported by:　　　　Signature:　　　　Date:		
What action was taken at the time? Reported by:　　　　Signature:　　　　Date:		
Any follow up action required and by whom?		
Level of risk attributed: None Minor Moderate Major Catastrophic		

Contributory factors: Environment ❑ Team ❑ Individual ❑ Patient ❑ Task ❑ Organisational ❑ Institutional context ❑	Notification/actions: Recorded in notes ❑ Patient notified ❑ Occupational Health notified ❑ Legal department notified ❑ Statutory body notified (such as HSE) ❑ Other ❑ ❑

This document is for quality assurance purposes only and should not be filed in any patients notes.

Who needs a form? 4.27

The example form in **FIGURE 4.2** includes a minimum data set and allows for some evaluation of what occurred. Any form will need a published procedure so that it is clear what information should be provided and why. This particular form is one side of A4 paper, but is self-carbonating in three parts for the following reasons:

- one part is retained in the ward or department as part of its own internal audit and review process;

- one is sent to the risk management or quality department for processing; and

- one is sent to another department or speciality that may have been involved.

An example which demonstrates the importance of the third copy is a dispensing error that is not picked up in pharmacy, but instead is picked up on the ward.

The form would be completed and the third copy sent to the pharmacy manager to assess practice and quality control as part of their internal review of incidents and procedures.

It is worth noting that the contributory factor categories used in the form are taken from the work of University College London and the Association of Litigation and Risk Managers, who have published a protocol for the investigation of clinical incidents.[3]

Tick boxes or free text?   4.28

One disadvantage of the sample form in **FIGURE 4.2** is that legibility can become an issue. If a form is used that has tick boxes for a host of potential incidents within different specialties, then the data form can be scanned and automatically entered into a database system. With free text forms, the information needs to be entered into a system manually. An example of how tick boxes can be used is shown in Table 4.1.

Table 4.1: Tick boxes

Specialty		Category of incident	
• Cardiac	☐	• Clinical (patient)	☐
• Medicine	☐	• Security	☐
• Clinical support	☐	• Staff incident	☐
• Surgery	☐	• Violence	☐
• Obstetrics	☐	• Drug/medication	☐
• Accident & Emergency	☐	• Other	☐
Type of incident		Specialty specific (acute)	
• Delay in diagnosis	☐	• Removal of wrong organ	☐
• Health records not available	☐	• Allergic reaction to drug	☐
• Adverse drug reaction	☐	• History not taken or checked	☐
• Defective medical device	☐	• Blood sample cross-matched for wrong patient	☐

Beware that when using a tick-box form it will need to be as inclusive as possible for those completing it. The reason for this is to avoid overuse of the 'other' category: it should not become the default category because the person completing the form cannot find the category or description they are looking for.

The form can also contain specialty-specific sections for mental health, ambulance services and primary care. Examples of primary care can be related to a number of services; for dental treatment, for example: the extraction of the wrong tooth; excessive bleeding following treatment; or death as a result of anaesthesia. For general practice: an unexpected death in the practice or clinic; abnormal cervical smears not reported to a patient; incorrect repeat prescriptions for a patient; and, again, delay in diagnosis.

The DoH form

4.29

The DoH has published a pilot incident report form, which is simple, confined to free text and contains some of the minimum data sets discussed earlier. To ensure confidentiality, patient details are confined to factors such as gender, age and ethnic group. Staff involved are granted anonymity; their designation is the only requirement.

Confidentiality

4.30

This approach provides the level of confidence required for a national reporting system. After all, it can be difficult enough to get healthcare staff to use an internal reporting system to its maximum advantage and, in so doing, feel safe in reporting. To step outside the organisation and report to the National Patient Safety Agency must be done in a manner that will ensure staff safety and security is maintained, even in this day and age of advanced healthcare and increased public scrutiny.

Grading incidents

4.31

The grading or categorisation of incidents is important as it provides information on the level of risk prevalent within a speciality, but it also allows the organisation to prioritise and concentrate on the key issues arising from reporting. As shown in the sample incident report form, five risk–grading categories are used: none, minor, moderate, major and catastrophic. The National Patient Safety Agency uses these definitions. How these are defined for impact and consequence is summarised in TABLE 4.2.

Table 4.2: Grading of incidents

Descriptor	Actual or potential impact	Numbers of persons actually or potentially affected	Actual or potential impact on organisation
Catastrophic	Death, including: • unexpected death whilst under the direct care of a health professional • death of a patient on GP or health centre premises • suicide or homicide by a patient being treated for a mental disorder • known or suspected case of healthcare associated infection which may result in death, such as hospital-acquired infection	• many (>50), eg. cervical screening concerns, vaccinations	• international adverse publicity/severe loss of confidence in the organisation • extended service closure • litigation >£1 million
Major	• major permanent harm • procedures involving the wrong patient or body part • haemolytic transfusion reaction • retained instruments or other material post-surgery requiring re-operation	• 16–50	• national adverse publicity/major loss of confidence in the organisation • temporary service closure • litigation £500–£1 million • increased length of stay >15 days

	• known or suspected case of healthcare associated infection which may result in permanent harm, such as hepatitis C • patient receiving a radiation dose whilst undergoing a medical exposure • rape (but only on determination that a rape has actually occurred, or the organisation believes there is significant evidence) • infant abduction, or discharge to the wrong family		• increased level of care >15 days
Moderate	• semi-permanent harm (up to one year), including: • known or suspected healthcare associated infection which may result in semi-permanent harm	• 3–15	• local adverse publicity or moderate loss of confidence • litigation £50,000–£500,000 • increased length of stay 8–15 days • increased level of care 8–15 days
Minor	• non-permanent harm (up to one month), including: • known or suspected healthcare associated infection which may result in non-permanent harm	• 1–2	• litigation <£50,000 • increased length of stay 1–7 days • increased level of care 1–7 days
None	• no obvious harm	• not applicable	• minimal impact, no service disruption

Establishing reporting as an everyday activity   4.32

Reporting is the operative word here for the assumption is made that all incidents are being reported, when in fact they are not. Therefore, the focus of activity is centred on a small proportion of reported incidents, with the unknown, hidden risks not being accounted for and therefore not being addressed

'Corridor conversations'   4.33

This is where informal personal networks of healthcare professionals become crucial, for they often indicate where there are particular incidents arising within the organisation. These informal networks, which might be termed 'corridor conversations', should be treated with confidence. However, if a serious risk is identified and it is substantiated by evidence, then it must be made clear to those who are aware of the incident that it must be reported through the appropriate reporting mechanisms. To ignore the incident could be a breach of duty of care of patients and a possible failure to comply with health and safety law. The *Public Disclosure Act 1998* makes it possible for individuals to raise concerns, but if the organisational culture is right, this should not have to be initiated through a whistle-blowing policy, even though it is right to have this policy in place.

Over reporting   4.34

The challenge is to make incident reporting an everyday activity even to the point of over-reporting. This will succeed in a culture that is open and honest about incidents, how they are reported and, more importantly, how they are dealt with and what lessons are learnt. To achieve this, there will be merit in having 'noise' in the system to begin with, through over-reporting, and then, through review and analysis of information, determining what the level of reporting *should* be. To do this will require a level of staffing that can cope with a high volume of reporting, provided the introduction of the incident reporting system is successful.

Reviewing incidents   4.35

'Review' of incidents is a positive term used for investigating an incident. The word suggests an approach that is open and transparent. 'Investigation' can often be taken to mean a harder-edged approach, even if it is not meant to be. Reviewing an incident fits in with the concept of risk and quality being interrelated making it a positive approach to improving care rather than a negative one.

This is not to say that a review cannot be firm in its approach and searching within the process adopted. The Commission for Health Improvement (CHI) has undertaken reviews, and published findings that have had some far-reaching implications for NHS organisations. Depending on the type of healthcare organisations involved, reviews can be quite a useful tool to understand the root causes of incidents, and develop learning for staff and patients.

The review process 4.36

In reviewing incidents, there must be an individual responsible for managing the review, whether at a local level or at a wider organisational one. Incidents that are defined as catastrophic or major will certainly require a review. This should apply to near-miss events, not just those with a known impact or outcome. There must also be a procedure about what information will need to be gathered, what should be retained and the legal status afforded to the review and subsequent documents and reports.

Spotting incident patterns 4.37

Normally a clinician or manager will undertake the initial review and in practice, senior managers get involved only if the incident is of such a serious nature that a wider review and analysis is required. An example of this would be the three incident rule, referred to earlier (see **4.2**), where an incident is repeated three times but not necessarily by the same people or department. This trend would only be picked up by senior managers who reviewed reported incidents in a particular speciality, or those who review the data from the organisation as a whole and see the pattern emerging. This takes a keen and experienced eye.

What the review examines 4.38

Incident reviews will encapsulate the reason or reasons why the incident occurred. This entails looking at the level of performance of those involved and the environment at the time. Root cause analysis or similar methodology can be applied to identify and understand the underlying causes, including those that have an organisational origin.

Reviews may be seen as time-consuming, but should nonetheless be recorded as part of the quality cycle of performance. Methods can be devised that make the process rigorous and thorough when it needs to be, but less thorough for low-risk incidents. One way to do this is by using the incident form as the review tool itself. Where a thorough approach is required, the use of an aide memoire or checklist can be used to guide staff through the process. For example:

- reviewing documentation;
- interviewing staff;
- obtaining statements; and
- meticulous note-taking.

Support for individuals 4.39

Where statements may be required, particularly if the incident may result in a potential claim, staff should be given the opportunity to have a representative involved such as a trade union official or personnel officer. The individual involved in the review should be well-supported and given access to essential information. In particularly traumatic events, NHS organisations should be able to call on immediate counselling or other support systems to help staff and indeed patients come to terms with what they have just experienced.

The report   4.40

At the end of the review process, a report should be produced that gives those involved an opportunity to comment on the findings. The report should:

●   be concise and outline the key points of the review with supporting recommendations;

●   reference key documents that support the findings and recommendations;

●   give guidance as to what future changes will be required;

●   provide a timetable for putting in proposed changes; and

●   outline who is responsible for ensuring that the changes are implemented.

All reports should form part of a quality assurance cycle. This way there is a method of accountability to make sure that recommendations are indeed acted upon. One way of doing this is through the workings of a clinical governance and risk management committee. This will in part ensure senior management and board-level responsibility for incidents and risk.

Analysing information   4.41

Analysing information can often be the most challenging part of a review as it can be difficult and confusing to draw conclusions. There may be too much information making it hard to discern what is important. Another reason may be the way the information is collated, which does not allow for particular patterns or trends to be identified.

Data should be looked at in the context of other information and not in isolation. Incident reporting should be seen as part of an information management system drawn from a range of sources and presented in a way that summarises the key issues and states assumptions where assumptions are made.

Analysing the data in context   4.42

The range of information sources that should be considered, compared and contrasted with data gathered from reported incidents is listed below. This list is not exhaustive, but gives a fair indication of information that can be used to obtain a picture of what is happening within the organisation. This includes:

- Complaints information – generated by patients themselves or their relatives (this information is often complementary to incidents, and indicates when incidents should have been reported through the incident reporting system rather than as a complaint).

- Review of medical records to establish any adverse events (usually through clinical audit cycles).

- Morbidity and mortality data and peer review information.

- Clinical audit reports and recommendations.

- Potential claims held within the organisation.

- Claims data held by the NHS Litigation Authority – this can be used as a benchmark for levels and types of claims and give an indication of where incident reporting may be weak or ineffective.

- Reports from sources such as the Health and Safety Executive and the National Audit Office.

- Regional information on critical adverse events notification and the National Patient Safety Agency.

- Stakeholders' views on the standard and quality of service.

- Assessments from the Clinical Negligence Scheme for Trusts.

- CHI and CHAI reviews.

Communications systems   4.43

Reviews of data in some healthcare organisations have shown that there is evidence of a correlation between incidents, complaints and claims but that to make effective use of the information, there must be good communication between people and services. If computer software systems are being used, it is preferable to either link these or use software that has the modules for each of these functions. That way one patient or employee database can be used, allowing an analysis of individuals as well as incidents.

Making the most of the data   4.44

So far the review of an incident has been considered on a case-by-case basis. From a departmental or speciality view, this is quite effective; but what do incidents say about the management of an organisation as a whole? The aggregation of data enables managers to determine what trends and patterns are occurring with reported incidents, and also provides a means of comparison with other organisations to determine what incidents are not being reported. It will be a requirement of the National Patient Safety Agency to provide incident information on a routine basis, excluding that required via their reporting form and system.

Essential functions of a data collection system   4.45

Whatever the data collection system used, certain information will need to be presented and commented upon. This is best achieved by using an electronic recording product, whether this involves commercial software or the development of an in-house database system. There are some essential functions that any system, even a manual one, must have if it is to provide useful management information.

These are:

- type of incident;
- number of incidents reported;
- contributory factors;
- risk grading;
- nature of the harm recorded; and
- location or speciality.

Type of incident   4.46

This will give information on what type of incidents were reported. For example, how many were classified as clinical incidents, how many were non-clinical (which would involve estates and facilities issues) and, importantly, how many were classified as near-misses. Each type of incident should then be capable of being broken down – for example, clinical incidents would be subdivided into categories such as anaesthetics, surgery, treatment and diagnosis. Therefore, the coding system used within the organisation must be well thought through and lend itself to providing useful and meaningful management information.

Number of incidents reported   4.47

Just like information on complaints presented to trust boards, incident information should also give basic information such as the number of incidents reported over a specified period of time. This is normally shown quarter by quarter. The data can then be compared against each subsequent quarter or compared to the same quarter of the previous year or earlier, as shown in **FIGURE 4.3**.

Figure 4.3: Number of incidents per quarter over three years

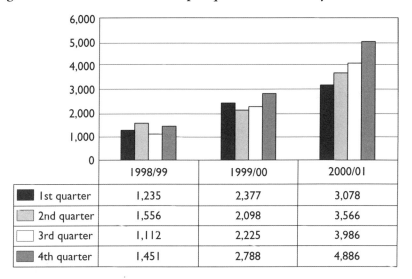

	1998/99	1999/00	2000/01
■ 1st quarter	1,235	2,377	3,078
▨ 2nd quarter	1,556	2,098	3,566
☐ 3rd quarter	1,112	2,225	3,986
▩ 4th quarter	1,451	2,788	4,886

Figure 4.3 demonstrates an increase in reported incidents year on year, with some fluctuation within the quarters of each year. This increase lends itself to various interpretations. One person may think that more incidents are occurring and thus there is an increase in risk within the organisation. However, another view may be that more incidents are being reported, but not necessarily occurring – in other words, staff are actually using the reporting system, one small indicator that it is successful.

That is not the full story, however, because the numbers alone are meaningless. If the numbers were then taken as a ratio against the number of finished consultant episodes (FCEs) or outpatient attendances, then they would become more meaningful. It would also be much easier to see if there is a true trend in upward or downward reporting and there would also be an indication of whether the activity of the hospital in this case has increased or decreased. The HSE produces annual accident statistics which are expressed in frequency rates, that is, numbers of accidents for so many employees. This enables comparison to be made on performance across sectors.

Contributory factors 4.48

Not only is it important to classify the type of incident and establish whether the numbers are on the increase or not, but it is important to understand, through coding, what the contributory factors may have been. Referring back to the sample incident form in **FIGURE 4.2**, these are shown in the bottom left hand corner of the form. These contributory factors are usually determined during the review stage of an incident, but in the case of the organisation that uses this form, they form part of the incident reporting procedure.

Contributory factors can be added to the breakdown of incidents reported in a medical directorate over a period of time (see **FIGURE 4.4**), but what is even better about using contributory factors as a data set for analysis is that they can be cross-tabulated with other data sets such as specialities, risk grading or immediate causes.

Figure 4.4: Contributory factors plotted against incident numbers

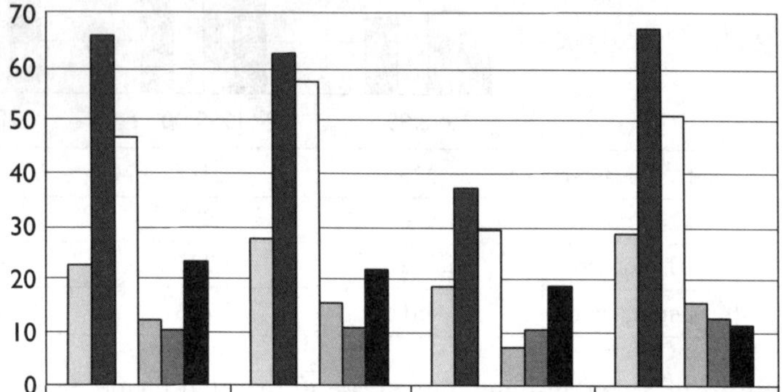

	1st quarter	2nd quarter	3rd quarter	4th quarter
Team	22	26	18	27
Patient	62	59	35	63
Individual	44	54	28	48
Organisation	12	15	7	15
Environment	10	11	10	12
Task	22	21	18	11

Risk grading
4.49

Working with the National Patient Safety Agency's recommendations and the risk grading shown in the sample incident report form in **FIGURE 4.2**, analysis of this data set is also of value. As a word of caution, however, (that should also be applied to contributory factor coding) the people applying the codes must be clear and consistent in the coding they use. If they are not then the data will not be useful, and can in fact skew the information in such a way that incidents requiring action are excluded.

Nature of the harm recorded
4.50

This will detail the injury sustained, if it is known at the time. This would include death, physical injury to parts of the body, pain, incapacity or disease.

Trend analysis 4.51

It is important to be able to break any recorded data down into the number and type of incidents reported by department, specialty or by practice, in the case of primary care. Comparisons can be made on a quarterly or other specified time frame and between specialties where there are common criteria, for example, the number of needlestick injuries sustained by nursing or medical staff or the number of back injuries reported. There must be caution applied when using this approach and a clear understanding of the criteria used to make comparisons. Any assumptions made must be clearly stated.

Other data sets can be used, such as incident costs, but these in the past have been often difficult to ascertain and use with consistency. There may also be an associated perception that incident reporting becomes more of a financial model for managing risk than a quality-driven one.

Electronic systems 4.52

Having electronic collection and analysis of data is by far the most preferable means of understanding incidents. To take this one step further, with the advancement of the NHS National Programme for IT, paper-based incident reporting systems will move to electronic systems over time.

The benefits of electronic entry include instant access to information and shortening the time of review and action, where needed. Such a system also gives clinical managers the ability to interrogate and analyse information from their own workplace, giving them the freedom and flexibility to be more proactive in managing risk in their own environment. Increased use of electronic-based systems also makes benchmarking easier.

Cross-analysis 4.53

In addition to the basic analysis of data, cross-tabulation allows the comparison of one data set against another to see if there are trends or patterns emerging. For example, contributory factors could be tabulated against a number of specialties to see if the individual factors were the most common factor involved in incidents reported. This would indicate, from an education and learning perspective, that support and supervision may be required in a number of areas. This can be broken down further to look at the professional groups involved.

Data recorded over time will bring the opportunity to map out trends. Cross-analysis will allow evaluation of clinical incidents on a month-by-month basis in one speciality, using the ratio figure rather than the raw numbers (see earlier discussion on the use of FCEs, SEE **4.47**) and identification of emerging trends. Good software packages or the application of the statistical analysis tools in a database package will calculate mean and standard deviation, regression lines and straight line extrapolations. The organisation will need to have people with good research and analytical skills in order to take this data, analyse it and present it as management information.

Learning lessons   4.54

Learning lessons from incidents cannot be discussed without reference to the significant work undertaken for *An Organisation with a Memory* (see **KEY REFERENCES, APPENDIX 1**). This document paints a picture of optimism in the face of traditional ways of working and an NHS culture requiring change to become more open and transparent as public bodies and, in so doing, accept accountability. The NHS must be willing and able to admit to mistakes when it needs to, and to learn lessons from events. The establishment of the National Patient Safety Agency is a clear signal that the NHS will listen and learn, both at a local as well as national level.

This is of course easier said than done. High profile cases such as the Bristol paediatric heart surgery scandal, which resulted in an intensive public inquiry (see also **CHAPTER 9**), and the Alder Hey Children's Hospital organ retention scandal have led the public to openly question the culture of the NHS, and rightly so. These messages are clear and strong ones that leaders in the NHS must be mindful of.

The seven steps to patient safety, as quoted from the NPSA's guidance, provide a concise approach for NHS staff to follow:

'Step 1 Build a safety culture – create a culture that is open and fair

Step 2 Lead and support your staff – establish a clear and strong focus on patient safety throughout your organisation

Step 3 Integrate your risk management activity – develop systems and processes that manage our reisks and identify and assess things that could go wrong

Step 4 Promote reporting – ensure staff can easily report incidents locally and nationally

Step 5 Involve and communicate with patients and the public – develop ways to communicate openly and listen to patients

Step 6 Learn and share safety lessons – encourage staff to use root cause analysis to learn how and why incidents happen

Step 7 Implement solutions to prevent harm – embed lessons through changes to practice, processes or systems.'

Readers are strongly encouraged to access the NPSA website: *www.npsa.nhs.uk* to gain an understanding of the seven step approach and the workings of the NPSA including the publication of patient safety alerts.

A proactive approach   4.55

A proactive approach to identifying what goes on in a healthcare organisation, irrespective of the size of the organisation, must be a good thing. The concept of size is important, because media focus is often on the treatment received in hospital, or on a handful of cases involving mentally ill individuals. Primary care, where the majority of first contact with the NHS takes place, receives little attention and it could be argued that the risks are just as significant: missed or delayed diagnosis, inappropriate treatment and care, medication errors to name a few.

Taking a proactive approach means that this must be led from within the organisation, asking people to champion the identification and reporting of incidents, making sure that the lessons are learnt that will improve the standard of care patients receive. The same holds true for staff safety and welfare.

Learning lessons across organisational boundaries   4.56

This leads to the consideration of learning lessons from incidents across NHS and social care boundaries. Both this chapter and **CHAPTER 2** imply that the systems to be put in place are only for a specific organisation, be it an acute care hospital, a doctor's surgery or a small community hospital. That is usually the case.

If the care provided is to be person–centred, then from the patient's perspective, who provides the care is irrelevant. What they are interested in is receiving the right treatment by the right people at the right time. If an incident occurs which disrupts the quality of that care, and if it occurs in more than one NHS organisation, how are the lessons learnt by all those involved? The answer is that at the moment, they are not.

With this in mind, this last and final section of this chapter will consider how lessons can be learnt, and, more importantly, that they must be learnt without the constraints of organisational boundaries.

Breaking down barriers   4.57

The first step is to recognise the barriers to learning. Once identified, these can then be broken down and removed in order that effective learning can indeed take place.

Recognising personal fallibility   4.58

The barriers to learning are many and they apply to a range of organisations and industries, the NHS being no exception. The difference for the NHS is that the professionals it employs have a duty of care to others, both ethically and legally, that they must comply with. One of the first barriers is the inability for professionals to recognise that they are fallible, can make mistakes and therefore have a need to improve their own practice and performance.

This first and profound barrier is actively being dealt with through professional bodies, but also by the Department of Health through the introduction of the NHS Plan (see KEY REFERENCES, APPENDIX 1) and the requirements that it imposes on professionals, from appraisal through to patient involvement and participation. Being accountable for our own actions and having the insight to recognise when standards have not been what we have aimed for are two behavioural changes that will need to occur within organisations, some of this being lead by example by practitioners themselves.

Ineffective communication   4.59

Another key barrier and undoubtedly one of the root causes of most incidents is ineffective communication within an organisation. This can be prevalent within clinical teams and at board level. Both can be damaging and can bar effective learning for many within an organisation. A risk management strategy, which will embrace the tool of incident reporting, should include how information will be shared with others and importantly, what changes have occurred as a result of reporting. This too needs to be communicated.

Lack of corporate responsibility   4.60

Not having a sense of corporate responsibility makes it difficult to implement changes in behaviour and changes in practice. This could be particularly true with independent contractors who may not feel any corporate responsibility to a primary care trust because of their status. However, the same lack of corporate responsibility can also be found in hospitals, where clinicians opt out of decisions taken by the organisation and carry on irrespective of what has been decided or implemented.

A sense of corporacy, acquired through the leadership of trust boards is one way of instilling a sense of corporate responsibility and leadership – of course, this is contingent upon the clinical and managerial leadership displayed within the organisation. trust boards can effectively demonstrate this by publishing incident data and findings of reports that don't breach patient confidentiality, but instead identify the key themes and the changes put in place to rectify them.

Outside the healthcare sector, it is fairly common for organisations to report on incidents in their annual report. Typical information included is:

- Enforcement action by enforcing authorities.
- *RIDDOR* notifications.
- Recorded incidents.
- Cases of ill health and sickness/absence.
- Results of audits.

CHI publishes the star ratings for NHS organisations each year, which are based on a range of performance indicators, one such indicator is sickness/absence. Information, as shown above, however is not reported. NHS organisations are required to produce, in their annual report, a Statement of Internal Control, that states the risks to the organisation and steps to manage such risks. This Statement might provide the opportunity for NHS organisations to report the type of information others outside the NHS currently provide.

Apportioning blame   4.61

Apportioning blame, a feature of inward-looking organisations with a very hierarchical and often dictatorial style, needs to be replaced with a culture based on learning. This requires leadership and very effective change management strategies employed over a period of time, and it may take years to see any demonstrable change. The time needed for this change, however, should not be an obstacle to dealing with the issue of blame. Using organisational development as a change agent to move an organisation to one of openness and honesty is recommended.

Individual reactions to criticism   4.62

The last barrier mentioned here (although there are more) is the difficulty that individuals have when faced with initiatives and the possibility that people will review and perhaps question their individual practice. Reactions to this vary, with some individuals finding it very difficult to listen to constructive criticism and others focusing on the process of incident reporting and the insignificant rather than the significant. The use of appraisal systems in a constructive, supportive atmosphere is an effective tool for change so that incidents are seen in the overall context of an individual's work, not separate from it.

A learning organisation   4.63

Learning is not simply about taking someone out of their environment for a training session, but using personal experience as part of overall learning within an organisation. In addition, education and research must be the foundation for building a learning organisation, one which can continuously move forward to improve care.

These may be fine words, but the challenge is putting them into practice. By using some of the practical points outlined within this chapter and drawing on the strategic overview of managing risk in **CHAPTER 2**, the foundation for learning can start to be applied, but this should be done in the context of other systems and procedures in place. There is a wealth of information available in healthcare settings and it is not used to its full effect.

Putting in a robust yet simple incident reporting system that can be integrated into operational activities is the first step, but it must be based on inclusion and consultation of staff. This way employees will feel they too have a stake in the system, are mindful to use it, and want it to be successful. Secondly, collecting the data in a clear and concise way and then presenting it as useful management information will allow the factors contributing to the incident to be exposed.

Taking this one stage further, aggregating the data and comparing and contrasting it both internally and externally, linking it with other information and devolving responsibility within the organisation to review incidents as part of a quality process will help achieve improvements and changes in practice.

Learning cannot be confined within the boundaries of one NHS organisation, but it must cross NHS and social care boundaries. If incidents are picked up in secondary care or social services that may have originated in primary care, then it is feasible to discuss the incident with those involved and seek action to ensure that the incident does not occur again. Learning should be done in a way that is not threatening and is seen as an aid to improve care, focusing on the patient rather than on the healthcare organisation and its individuals.

References

1   Department of Health (2002) *Building a Safer NHS for Patients.*
2   Department of Health (2001) *Doing Less Harm.*
3   University College London & Association of Litigation and Risk Management (ALARM), *A protocol for the investigation of clinical incidents*, Royal Society of Medicine Press, London, 1999.

Further information

See also KEY REFERENCES, piii

Burrows, M (1997), 'Incident reporting and performance management', *The Healthcare Risk Resource*, Vol 1, no 2.

Department of Health (2001), *A Commitment to Quality, a Quest for Excellence*, (*www.doh.gov.uk*)

Health and Safety Executive (1997), HSG 65, *Successful health and safety management*, (*www.hse.gov.uk*)

Tingle, J (2000), 'The report that rocked a nation', *Health Care Risk Report,* Vol 6, no 8, pp 20–21.

Useful websites

www.hse.gov.uk

www.npsa.nhs.uk

www.doh.gov.uk

www.chi.org

Chapter 5
Clinical Risk Management: Law, Policy and Context

This chapter covers:

- Clinical negligence litigation.

- Role of National Health Service Litigation Authority (NHSLA).

- Clinical Negligence Scheme for Trusts (CNST).

- Clinical risk management standards.

- Role of Commission for Healthcare Audit and Inspection (CHAI).

- Clinical governance.

- Role of the National Patient Safety Agency (NPSA).

- Reform of the clinical negligence system.

Introduction   5.1

In this chapter clinical risk management will be discussed within the context of a number of NHS care quality improvement initiatives. Key aspects of the NHS quality improvement infrastructure will be covered along with issues relating to clinical negligence litigation.

This chapter will show that clinical risk management and clinical negligence are related. Through the proper application of clinical risk management strategies clinical negligence litigation should be avoided or at least exposure to it minimised. Looking at the healthcare environment realistically and the high number of care episodes carried out daily in the NHS it will never be possible to totally eliminate the possibility of adverse or negligent acts occurring. Human nature dictates that they will happen, the key is to make them happen less and to minimise their outcome. The National Patient Safety Agency (NPSA) recognises the inevitability of some mistakes being made:

> 'Every day more than a million people are treated safely and successfully in the NHS. But the evidence tells us that in complex healthcare systems things will and do go wrong, no matter how dedicated and professional the staff. And when things do go wrong, patients are at risk of harm.'[1]

95

The problem of clinical negligence litigation   5.2

Clinical negligence litigation has been with us for quite some time, first becoming a noticeable problem around 1978, although its existance can be seen in case law reports well before then. An early and valuable discussion on the topic can be found in Ham et al's discussion of medical negligence and compensation and accountability in 1988.

The author's state:

> 'Various explanations have been proposed for the growth over the last decade in litigation arising from medical accidents ... we do not think it is plausible simply to attribute the increase in litigation to a direct copying of American experience. Three other types of explanation have been put forward: a real increase in negligence; easier access to legal representation; and a change in the propensity of patients to sue following an adverse outcome.'[2]

Whatever the exact date, the issue remains that clinical negligence and avoiding it has been a serious problem for over 25 years and the issues highlighted by Ham et al are as current and fresh now as they were back in 1988.

Ham et al conclude:

> '... consideration needs to be given to a range of other policy options designed to encourage high quality medical care. In the short term, the most promising options worth pursuing are those which aim to strengthen professional accountability ... regardless of whether or not a system of no fault compensation is introduced, a strong case can be made for improving complaints procedures, reforming the procedures used to discipline doctors, and encouraging the extension of medical audit.'

All these recommendations can be seen to have been adopted although clinical audit never seemed to be fully embraced within the NHS.

The NHS has clearly changed considerably since the late 1970s and 1980s, it has more resources and there are more patients to treat for a greater number of conditions. However, the problem of what to do about increasing clinical negligence litigation claims and costs has always remained constantly in the shadows. With the publication of *Making Amends*[3] there is now a real opportunity to fully address this issue.

Clinical negligence litigation today   5.3

The cost and frequency of clinical negligence claims and complaints about clinical care have been increasing for a number of years. The National Audit Office (NAO)[4] state that the rate of new claims per thousand finished consultant episodes rose by 72% between 1990 and 1998.

An idea of the costs of clinical negligence were given in *Making Amends:*[3]

'Comprehensive information on the costs of claims and compensation paid for clinical negligence has not until recently been collected centrally by the NHS.

Data from the NHS Litigation Authority (established in 1995), surveys of NHS Trust hospitals commissioned for this report and earlier 'one off' surveys and estimates show that:

- annual NHS clinical negligence expenditure rose from £1 million in 1974/75 … to £446 million in 2001/02;

- claimants' legal costs outweigh defendant's legal costs; for cases settled with an award in 2002/03 they were 82% higher for older cases and 88% higher for more recent cases;

- the National Audit Office found that the legal and administrative costs of settling claims exceed the money actually paid to the victim in the majority of claims under £45,000 and take up an even higher proportion of smaller claims.'

In discussing future NHS liability for clinical negligence the report states:

'Estimates from research conducted for this report, based on a larger sample of 136 NHS Trusts, gave a broadly similar result. That reported just under 22,000 outstanding claims at April 2001, with an estimated value of nearly £5.6 billion.'

The Health Service Ombudsman (HSO) annual reports frequently note an increase of complaints over the previous year and the latest is no exception.[5]

A key issue resulting from the above discussion is what to do about clinical negligence litigation and complaints. These factors are all linked together with the management of clinical risk and securing quality health care services. They all form part of the same circle. The increasing costs, numbers of cases and complaints have caused concern in all quarters. The response of the Government has been to create a succession of health quality improvement, regulatory initiatives and agencies to address the problem.

Litigation against the NHS has now become centrally managed by the National Health Service Litigation Authority (NHSLA).

Improving healthcare quality in the NHS: A proliferation of quangos   5.4

Since the publication of Ham et al's report[2] a number of new bodies have been established to tackle the problem of quality of patient care by improving the management of clinical risk and introducing best practice.

The functions of some of these agencies are below (SEE **5.8**) in this chapter and elsewhere in this book.

Organisations such as National Institute for Clinical Excellence (NICE), Commission for Health Improvement (CHI), Commission for Healthcare Audit and Inspection (CHAI), National Health Service Litigation Authority (NHSLA) and the National Patient Safety Agency (NPSA) exist in order to achieve these objectives. They aim to ensure the delivery of high quality healthcare services. These organisations have an immense impact on the day to day working practices of NHS staff and in turn the experiences of NHS patients. As each organisation is created another healthcarer or manager accountability mechanism seems to be created. These organisations have a range of missions and agendas which may not necessarily coincide with each other.

To understand risk and litigation in the NHS, an understanding of the organisations that pepper the wide NHS landscape is needed. It is however becoming increasingly difficult for healthcare workers and those who advise them to become able to comprehend in any detail the function and purpose of all the agencies that currently exist in order to reform the NHS and implement Government health policy plans. According to Bennett[6] NHS hospitals are answerable to 36 separate regulators forcing them to spend millions of pounds on even more administrators to navigate their way through the system. According to Sherman:

'The number of health quangos, which cost the taxpayer £2.2 Billion, will be slashed as part of a wider onslaught on NHS bureaucracy.'[7]

The Health Secretary has ordered a review of the health quangos.

Sherman also states:

'There is also an overlap between the National Patient Safety Agency and the Commission for Patient Public Involvement in Health both of which safeguard patient standards.'

The NHS Reviews Coordination Group (RCG)[8] is also concerned about the number of NHS regulatory reviews, inspections and audits. It argues that the review system has grown by accretion and has resulted in duplication and overlap and that there is a lack of effective coordination between the many organisations, which carry out the reviews.

The NHS RCG report reveals some deep rooted problems with NHS quality regulation:

'Many of the problems that the survey illustrates have deep rooted causes that will take time to resolve. They result from:

● the lack of a leader among reviewing bodies which can coordinate and direct the overall review effort

- statutory requirements which sometimes prevent reviewing organisations from relying on other's work and sharing of information between reviewing bodies.

- different values and approaches of reviewing bodies

- different remits and focus of each reviewing body and a lack of knowledge about, and understanding of, others roles.

The creation of CHAI with a role to lead inspection of healthcare is a significant opportunity to start to resolve some of these deep-rooted problems.'

It is refreshing to see a more general awareness developing of the fact that the landscape of NHS quality and accountability mechanisms is cluttered and needs urgent simplification.

A period of organisational consolidation is needed and it will be interesting to see how well the quangos can work together and whether some become incorporated into others. They face a tough challenge in changing an ingrained NHS culture which has traditionally functioned in the reactive mode of 'coping'.

In considering the organisational landscape of clinical risk it is also important to note the political focus and emphasis of the Government's health quality reforms and the organisations that are charged with effecting initiatives that enhance the quality of patient care. The focus and prime directive of Government policy is firmly rooted in the patient as the prime factor in the care equation.

The patient is king in the new NHS   5.5

The clinical negligence system and NHS risk management processes exist within a healthcare policy context which puts the patient firmly at the centre of the NHS. This is evident from a number of DoH policy documents. The conventional wisdom shared by the Government and many in the NHS is that the NHS is a 1940's system operating in a 21st century world. The former Health Secretary Alan Milburn stated:

'The NHS today lives too much in the shadow of its own history; as an organisation where Government provided limited resources, doctors were left in charge of providing limited services and patients were expected to be grateful for the limits of what they received'.[9]

Government policy now dictates that the patient is the most important person in the NHS and that the service should revolve around their interests and not solely around those who run and work in it. Patient empowerment is the order of the day.[10]

The concept of a patient centered NHS can be seen as a recurrent theme in health quality policy initiatives but the Judges also have woken up to the idea that the NHS needs a culture change.

Lord Woolf's speech   5.6

Lord Woolf has ably summarised the issues of medical accountability and the role of the courts:

> ' ... until recently the courts treated the medical profession with excessive deference, but recently the position has changed. It is my judgment that it has changed for the better.'

He went on to say:

> 'The over deferential approach is captured by the phrase; 'Doctor knows best'. The contemporary approach is a more critical approach. It could be said that Doctor knows best if he acts reasonably and logically and gets his facts right.'

Lord Woolf also mentioned the medical scandals:

> 'The "automatic presumption of beneficence" has been dented by a series of well-publicised scandals. The Judges were not oblivious of these scandals. The deterioration in confidence by the public and Judges alike is evidenced by an increase of more than 30% in the number of complaints made to the General Medical Council.'[11]

The medical scandals of recent years   5.7

The highly publicised medical scandals of recent years, Shipman, Bristol, Alder Hay and gynaecologist Rodney Ledward[12] have lead to a greater patient and Government focus on medical discipline and medical performance. The conventional wisdom shared by many commentators in clinical negligence litigation and risk management is that today's patients are much more inquiring and demanding and less deferential than they once were. These scandals have helped push patients to this position.

Clinical risk organisations   5.8

The NHS organisations that feature in the clinical risk landscape will now be discussed and key relevant aspects of their work relevant to risk managers will be explored.

NHSLA   5.9

The National Health Service Litigation Authority (NHSLA) is a key organisation which maintains various functions described in a NHLSA fact sheet[13] as being:

' ...

(i)   To ensure claims are dealt with consistently and with due regard to the proper interests of the NHS and its patients.

(ii)   To manage the financial consequences of such claims and to advise the Department of Health of the likely future costs.

(iii) To advise the Department of Health on both specific and general issues arising out of claims against the NHS.

(iv)   To manage and raise the standards of risk management throughout the NHS.

(v)   To assist NHS bodies to comply with the Human Rights Act by providing a central source of information on relevant case-law development.'

The NHSLA is responsible for handling clinical negligence claims made against NHS trusts, Strategic Health Authorities (StHAs), Primary Care Trust's (PCTs) and the former Regional Health Authorities (RHAs).

They have an expert panel of solicitors located around the country which work with these organisations and the NHSLA. The NHSLA schemes are organised with clinical claims arising out of incidents occurring after 1 April 1995 being handled under the 'Clinical Negligence Scheme for Trusts' (CNST) which is a voluntary risk-pooling scheme for NHS trusts and PCTs.[14] Claims relating to incidents from before April 1995 are handled under the 'Existing Liabilities Scheme' (ELS), which is funded centrally by the DoH. There is a third much smaller scheme, the Ex-RHAs Scheme which covers clinical negligence claims against the Regional Health Authorities which were abolished in 1996.

Non-clinical claims are handled under the Liabilities to Third Parties Scheme (LTPS) and the Property Expenses Scheme (PES). The collective name for these two schemes is the Risk Pooling Scheme for Trusts (RPST) and claims relating to incidents arising after 1 April 1999 (or incidents arising after the NHS body joined the schemes, if that was later) are covered.

In 2002/3 the NHSLA received 7,798 claims under its clinical negligence schemes and 3,667 claims in respect of its non-clinical schemes.[14]

The CNST and its clinical risk management standards   5.10

The CNST has been around now for ten years and its clinical risk management standards have been refined and developed over this period. Prior to this scheme clinical risk management and risk management generally was an unknown entity to many trusts, sadly today some trusts still find difficulty applying the principles, a point explored later in this chapter. The CNST clinical risk management standards are stated in the CNST General Risk Management Manual:[15]

- **Standard 1: Learning from Experience: The trust proactively uses internal and external information to improve clinical care.**

  This standard focuses on how the trust ensures that lessons are learnt and patient care is improved through the effective reporting of adverse incidents and near misses in health care. This standard also considers external confidential reviews and lessons learnt from claims and complaint handling.

- **Standard 2: Response to major clinical incidents: There is a policy for the rapid follow-up of major clinical incidents.**

  This standard states that the policy must be clear and simple in order to ensure a rapid response. The responsible person needs to be sufficiently senior for decision making and the policy must cover arrangements for managing incidents which happen 'out of hours'.

- **Standard 3: Advice and Consent: Appropriate information is provided to patients on the risks and benefits of the proposed treatment or investigation, and the alternatives available, before a signature on a consent form is sought.**

  This standard requires that leaflets and other printed material should be provided to patients well before the proposed treatment, informing them about their condition, and the proposed treatment. The responsibility for the review and approval of written information for the patients should be clearly defined. The CNST assessor will expect to see leaflets from a range of the trust's specialities and activities.

- **Standard 4: Health Records: A comprehensive system for the completion, use, storage and retrieval of health records is in place. Record keeping standards are monitored through the clinical audit process.**

  This standard states that in order to achieve maximum points in the assessment the trust will need to demonstrate that there is one record per patient. If, however, more than one record exists then either:

  o   All records are automatically available at the first new patient consultation; or

  o   A resumé of key clinical factors is held in all sets of records.

- **Standard 5: Induction, Training and Competence: There are management systems in place to ensure the competence and appropriate training of all clinical staff.**

  This standard expects that all new staff regardless of grade or profession should receive a formal induction to the trust. Full points are awarded if specialists, career grades, consultants, registrars or other doctors starting out of rotation receive induction. The induction programme for clinical staff in training needs to address corporate issues. A record of formal induction training for consultants and records of attendance are required to be maintained for all staff. There must also be a systematic follow up of non-attendees.

- **Standard 6: Implementation of Clinical Risk Management: A clinical risk management system is in place.**

  This standard states that the full benefits of clinical risk management will only be obtained if there is a comprehensive and co-ordinated system and a positive support for it throughout the trust. It seeks to look at 'the sum of the parts' to assess how the individual components of the strategy, and the people involved, work together to achieve the objectives.

- **Standard 7: Clinical Care: There are clear procedures for the management of general clinical care.**

  This standard states that the public has a reasonable expectation that clinical staff are competent to perform their duties and learn from the errors in the past and that recent large-scale incidents have dented public confidence. This standard relates to selected areas of clinical care, and incorporates advice and direction from relevant authoritative bodies such as National Confidential Enquiries, the Royal Colleges and the DoH.

- **Standard 8: The Management of Care in Trusts Providing Mental Health Services: There are clear systems for the protection of the public and service users.**

  This standard recognises that there have been many instances of harm being caused to the public, to service users, and to staff, as a result of failure to design, implement and monitor practical systems. All trusts providing Mental Health Services, should be able to demonstrate that they have working systems in place to ensure that vulnerable service users receive full professional assessment leading to appropriate support, supervision and control during their care and on discharge.

- **Standard 9: Ambulance Service: There are clear procedures for the management of clinical risk in trusts providing Ambulance Services.**

  This standard states that the increasing contribution of clinical care by ambulance staff requires some areas of uncertainty to be clarified. This standard comprises criteria suggested by Ambulance trusts to facilitate the planned and co-ordinated delivery of patient care.

These CNST standards are not intended for use by PCTs or Ambulance Services (unless seeking accreditation at level 2 or 3 during 2003–2004). Separate standards designed to address the specific risks faced by these organisations and which bring together the requirements of the CNST and RPST standards have been developed.

NHS trusts pay a contribution towards the costs of litigation which is assessed actuarially in advance each year. The NHSLA will give discounts to trusts who comply with the CNST risk management standards and to those trusts with a good claims history. There are a number of CNST levels which trusts can progressively reach from 0–3. Those which achieve level 1 in all areas achieve a 10% reduction in their CNST contribution, achievements at level 2 brings a 20%

reduction. Reaching level 3 results in a 30% discount; very few trusts have attained this level.

CNST level attainment is also used as a performance indicator for Star Ratings and CHI. There are therefore direct financial incentives for trusts to excel at the CNST levels. Risk management assessment visits by CNST assessors take place at least once every two years in each member trust. The visits are used to check compliance with the risk management standards.

RPST 5.11

The RPST risk management standard (August 2003) contains criteria identical to the DoH's Controls Assurance core risk management standard. 'This standard aims to ensure that each NHS organisation, as part of its system of internal control, embeds a rigorous risk management process that covers all risks'.[13] To comply with this standard trusts have to meet the following criterions.[16] Each criterion is scored out of 100%:

- Criterion 1: Corporate and Individual Accountability for Managing Risk
- Criterion 2: Risk Management Strategy
- Criterion 3: Risk Management Organisational Structure
- Criterion 4: Incident Reporting and Management
- Criterion 5: Complaints and Claims Reporting and Management
- Criterion 6: Risk Management Process
- Criterion 7: Risk Management Training
- Criterion 8: Independent Assurance.

NHS trust contributions to the scheme can be reduced if it meets the requirement of the RPST Risk Management Standard as listed above. The discount levels are the same as those for the CNST.

The CNST and RPST standards provide a directing focus to trusts to implement good organisational frameworks and working practices essential for high quality patient care and the management of risk.

The NHSLA maintain other clinical risk management standards for maternity services, ambulance services and PCTs. There is also a surgical patient pathway and during 2003–2004 work is being done to develop a specific set of CNST clinical risk management standards for mental health and learning disabilities services.[13]

Is clinical risk management working: The impact of the CNST?   5.12

Experience suggests that clinical risk management is working in practice to improve the quality of patient care in trusts; but it is difficult without definitive outcome measurements to say precisely that this is the case. If trust staff, and organisations communicate more effectively and there is more reflective and evidence-based practice then, that must lead to care improvements, as a matter of sound common-sense at the very least. What is clear is that many trusts still find implementing clinical risk management strategies and general risk management initiatives difficult. These schemes have to compete with other DoH initiatives and that could mean that they are pushed down the priority scale of some trusts. Risk management is a component part of clinical governance and is assessed by CHI and from 1 April 2004 CHAI.

CHI View   5.13

CHI published a report on emerging themes from 175 clinical governance reviews[17] and some related to risk management. CHI found that many trusts are poor at managing potential risks to patients. Many staff fear reprisals if they reported things going wrong. The risks to patients are also made worse by staff shortages and poor attendance on mandatory training courses.

NHSLA view   5.14

The NHSLA[18] has expressed disappointment at the number of trusts assessed at level 0 by CNST assessors and are working actively with these trusts in the hope that they will soon achieve at least level 1 accreditation. The NHSLA[18] provide some figures on trust CNST and RPST attainment levels as at 31 March 2003:

CNST	
Total Number of Trust Members	277
Level 0	53
Level 1	177
Level 2	41
Level 3	4
No Score	2

RPST	
Failed	156
Passed	97
Not assessed	24

These figures speak for themselves, most trusts after ten years are still only at CNST level one and the next highest number achieved no level. Well over half of the trusts failed the RPST assessment.

The NHSLA, CNST manual[19] describe the basis of the levels:

> 'Level 1 criteria represent the basic elements of a clinical risk management framework.

> Levels 2 and 3 are more demanding. Many are concerned with the implementation and integration into practice of policies and procedures, monitoring them and acting on the results. These levels also require staff to have a good understanding of clinical risk issues'.

Worryingly 53 trusts out of 277 have no basic elements of risk management in place worthy of assessment at level 1. The RPST figures also present a worrying picture.

NAO view   5.15

The National Audit Office (NAO)[20] also considered the issue of trust compliance with clinical risk management standards and noted some major barriers to it.

Lack of resources (at two thirds of trusts); the culture, behaviour, or attitudes of staff of the organisation (at a third of trusts); and a lack of strategy, processes, or co-ordination (a quarter).They also noted that CHI have commented that some organisations had a culture that was not conducive to reporting risks.

All however is not doom and gloom on this front.

Progress and concern   5.16

The NAO state[20] that trusts have made some progress with the CNST and that some trusts have made some progress since May 2001, but that one in five have not achieved any level, and most have yet to move beyond level 1. However, 81% of trusts reported that they made changes following their CNST risk management assessment. Almost half had changed policies and procedures such as incident reporting and equipment maintenance. Others made changes in areas like health records management (20%) and patient consent procedures (10%); and had increased training and development activity particularly related to risk management (24%). About a quarter were working towards the next higher level of assessment.

It is reassuring to see that trusts are making some effort after the CNST assessments, what gives cause for concern however is that three quarters of the trusts seem content not to work towards the next CNST level. This attitude may be borne out of complacency and that they have achieved a certain 'comfort level' given their resources and other competing priorities. Trusts should focus on attaining the next level as a show, at the very least, of their commitment to improving patient care; they owe it to their patients to improve.

Where the claims are: specialities 5.17

The NHLSA[18] provide some facts and figures on the number of reported CNST claims by speciality which is helpful as it can provide a focus of where to direct clinical risk management strategies and scarce resources:

Speciality	Claims
Surgery	6497
Obstetrics and Gynaecology	3863
Medicine	2740
Accident and Emergency	1722
Psychiatry/Psychology/Mental Health	448
Anaesthesia	432
Pathology	309
Radiology	291
Paramedical Support Services	156
Ambulance	138
Public Health	59
Primary Care (GP)	22
Nursing	14

CHAI 5.18

The Commission for Healthcare Audit and Inspection (CHAI) comes into effect on 1 April 2004. CHAI replaces CHI which will close. CHAI will build upon the work done by CHI and a number of other organisations.

CHAI's function will be to enhance the quality of healthcare by providing an independent assessment of the standards of service provided to patients, whether it is provided by the NHS or privately.

CHAI functions also include:

• providing an independent assessment of complaints;

• assessing the arrangements in place to promote public health; and

• acting as the leading inspectorate in relation to healthcare.[21]

A key practical focus of CHAI's work is to enhance and secure quality healthcare provision through its clinical governance inspections. The Clinical Governance Reviews previously undertaken by CHI will be replaced by CHAI over a period of time with new approaches to inspection and assessment.[22]

CHI review   5.19

A CHI review looks at the effectiveness of the NHS organisation's clinical governance arrangements. It assesses the management provision and quality of service provided by the organisation. CHI will identify best practice which it will share with the rest of the NHS and areas for improvement.[23]

Clinical governance   5.20

CHI defines clinical governance as:[23]

> 'the system of steps and procedures adopted by the NHS to ensure that patients receive the highest possible quality of care. It includes
>
> • a patient centered approach
>
> • an accountability for quality
>
> • ensuring high standards of safety
>
> • improvements in patient services and care.'

Figure 5.1: CHI's model for clinical governance (Assessing Clinical Governance)[24]

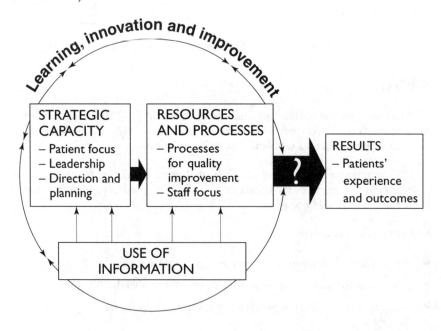

Figure 5.2: Components of clinical governance – resources and processes and use of information[24]

	Component
Resources and processes	
(i) process for quality improvement	Patient and public involvement
	Clinical audit
	Risk management
	Clinical effectiveness programmes
(ii) staff focus	Staffing and staff management
	Education, training and continuing professional and personal development
Use of information	Use of information to support clinical governance and health care delivery

CHI's review teams assess how well clinical governance is working by making enquiries about each of the seven components in Figure 5.2 at corporate and directorate levels and in clinical teams. On the basis of the evidence collected CHI reviewers assess each component against a four point scale.[24]

(1) Little or no progress at strategic and planning level, or at operational level

(2) (a) Worthwhile progress and development at strategic and planning levels but not at operational level; or

    (b) Worthwhile progress and development at operational level but not at strategic and planning levels; or

    (c) Worthwhile progress and developments at strategic and planning levels and at operational level but not across the whole organisation

(3) Good strategic grasp and substantial implementation. Alignment across the strategic and planning level, and the operational level of the trust

(4) Excellence – coordinated activity and development across the organisation and with partner organisations in the local health economy that is demonstrably leading to improvement. Clarity about the next stage of clinical governance.

Following a CHI review a report of the review team's findings is drafted and discussed with the NHS organisation under review for comments on factual accuracy. It is then published and is available both to the NHS organisation and to the public. The trust then produces an action plan to deal with the issues identified in the report. The relevant StHA or the Welsh Assembly Government approve the trust action plan and are responsible for ensuring its implementation.[24] The CHI clinical governance review, along with the trust's level of compliance against CNST risk management standards are performance indicators for the NHS performance star ratings for 2003–2004 as stated earlier.

Trusts therefore have clear incentives to improve the quality of patient care.

Themes for CHI clinical governance reviews   5.21

The CHI report[25] on emerging themes from 175 clinical governance reviews, the bulk of which were acute trusts, was mentioned in relation to the discussion of clinical risk management above.

The report also found some other themes:

'In more than 80% of NHS organisations reviewed the following themes emerged:

- NHS organisations are reactive rather than proactive-they respond to problems when they happen rather than anticipate them and so potentially avoid them

- There is a lack of organisation wide policies. In many cases, where policies do exist, they are not implemented or different departments have different policies on the same issue

- Learning is not shared between and across organisations

- Communication is not effective and there is a lack of sharing from strategic to operational levels, for example between senior mangers and those providing services, or between doctors and nurses.'

The findings also show that of the seven components of clinical governance, four are likely to cause concern. These are:

- Risk management.
- Staffing and staff management.
- Patient involvement.
- Use of information.

This is quite a damning catalogue of trust failings which calls for urgent attention and correction.

NAO and clinical governance   5.22

The NAO clinical governance report[20] was considered above in relation to the CNST clinical risk management standards. The NAO report considered other issues as well and found: that the clinical governance initiative has had many beneficial impacts that clinical quality issues are now more mainstream and there is a greater or more explicit accountability of both clinicians and managers for clinical performance. There is also evidence of improvements in practice and patient care, though trusts lack robust means of assessing this and overall progress.

The clinical governance initiative can be seen to have enhanced the profile of health care quality improvement initiatives and clinical risk management.

Along the way it has also tried to change a fairly ingrained NHS culture which instinctively seems to resist change. The NHS culture can be seen to be changing, albeit at a fairly slow pace. The NAO report shows that the very basic foundations of clinical governance can be seen to be in place in most trusts but that a lot more needs to be done.

The National Patient Safety Agency (NPSA)   5.23

An organisation that also expects healthcare quality improvement and improved patient safety is the National Patient Safety Agency (NPSA).

Running parallel with the CNST, NHSLA, CHI, CHAI and the clinical governance initiative is the NPSA. The NPSA was created in July 2001 to coordinate the efforts of the NHS in regard to patient safety. It provides a number of patient safety tools and the National Reporting and Learning System (NRLS).The NRLS is a patient safety incident data collection system which operates in the NHS.

There is some overlap of functions with all of the above organisations as they are all concerned with patient safety to some extent. The NPSA and the national patient safety initiative owes its existence largely to the seminal report[26] on patient safety in the NHS, 'An organisation with a memory', known colloquially as OWAM.

This report set the scene for subsequent patient safety initiatives and stands as an important source of information on what can go wrong in healthcare and how to stop it going wrong. The report gives some important insight into the patient safety problems in the NHS whilst also acknowledging that NHS reporting and information systems provide only a patchy and incomplete picture of the nature and scale of the problem of serious failures in healthcare. The report states that research evidence suggests that an estimated 850,000 (range 300,000 to 1.4 million) adverse events might occur each year in the NHS hospital sector, resulting in a £2 billion direct cost in additional hospital days. Some adverse events will be inevitable complications of treatment but around half might be avoidable. Over 6,600 adverse incidents involving medical devices were reported to the Medical Devices Agency in 1999, including 87 deaths and 345 serious injuries. Experience from the serious incident reporting system run by one of the NHS Executive's Regional Offices suggest that nationally at least 2,500 adverse events a year occur which should be serious enough to register on such systems. The cost to the NHS of hospital acquired infections have been estimated at nearly £1 billion a year, and around 15% of cases are regarded as preventable.

As well as highlighting the nature and scale of the problem of patient safety in the NHS the report looked at learning from failures and the evidence and experience from these. Conclusions drawn include:

- Awareness of the nature, causes and incidences of failures is a vital component of prevention - (You can't know what you don't know);

- Analysis of failures needs to look at root causes, not just proximal events; human errors cannot sensibly be considered in isolation of wider processes and systems.

- Error reduction and error management systems can help prevent or mitigate the effects of individual failures.

- Organisational learning is a cyclical process, and all the right components must be in place for effective, active learning to take place ....

- It is possible to identify a number of important barriers to learning ...

- Culture is a crucial component in learning effectively from failures ...

- Sound safety information systems are a precondition for systematic learning from failures. A number of key recommendations were made which included introducing a mandatory reporting system for adverse health care events and specified near misses. The encouragement of a reporting and questioning culture in the NHS and acting to ensure that important lessons are implemented quickly and consistently.[26]

This report was followed by another, *Building a Safer NHS for Patients*[27] where the Government set out its plans for promoting patient safety. The report focused on the local and national action needed to establish a system which ensures that lessons from adverse lessons from one locality are learnt across the whole NHS. The report lead to the creation of the NPSA.

Seven steps to patient safety   5.24

NPSA activity came to a peak in 2003 with the publication of its document, *Seven steps to patient safety*[1] where a series of measures designed to improve patient safety in the NHS were launched. The measures are commendable, exciting and maintain a real potential to improve patient safety in the NHS. What is less clear however is how they all fit and mesh together with the other patient safety initiatives such as the CNST and others described in this chapter. This point will be discussed further below. The NPSA have developed a simple checklist for NHS staff so that they can assess their progress towards delivering safer care.

The Seven Steps to Patient Safety
1.   Build a safety culture
2.   Lead and support your staff
3.   Integrate your risk management activity
5.   Promote reporting
5.   Involve and communicate with patients and the public
6.   Learn and share safety lessons
7.   Implement solutions to prevent harm

The NPSA further discuss these steps and the resources they will make available for them. Resources include a patient safety induction video, patient safety e-learning programme, safety culture survey, incident decision tree, National Reporting and Learning System (NRLS), root cause analysis training, root cause analysis tool, a network of patient safety managers.

Dealing with overlaps   **5.25**

There is a practical need when discussing the NPSA's *Seven steps to patient safety* report[1] to highlight important areas of overlap with other advice coming from NHS organisations such as the NHSLA, CHI and CHAI. Patient safety is clearly a key component of clinical risk management and it therefore links in with the CNST and the NHSLA.Clinical risk management is also an important aspect of clinical governance and therefore a clear link is made with CHI and CHAI.

No one health regulatory organisation has a monopoly over the concept but there does need to be some joined up thinking and co-ordination of endeavour going on. In Step 3 of Seven Steps there is no mention of the CNST.

The advice given in this step includes:

'Local risk management systems are designed to help NHS organisations manage incidents effectively and reduce the chances of them happening again. Patient safety is a key component of risk management, and should be integrated with staff safety, complaints management, litigation and claims handling, and financial and environmental risk. Local risk management systems should also be supported by an organisational risk management strategy, a programme of proactive risk assessments and the compilation of an organisation-wide risk register.'

The NPSA also advise on the setting up of local forums to discuss risk management and patient safety and to provide feedback to the relevant management groups. Some cross reference to the CNST and to the DoH controls assurance guidance would have been particularly helpful so that NHS staff and organisations could make the links and maintain more of a holistic, cross NHS overview of issues.

Step 5 could also have usefully benefited from a cross reference to CNST clinical risk management standards, particularly Standard 3 Advice and Consent.

The NPSA report states in Step 5 advice for organisations on apologies:

'acknowledge and apologise for failings in the care they deliver, and reassure patients and their families that the right lessons have been learnt from patient safety incidents.'

Such advice is commendable and is reflective of the sentiments expressed in *Making Amends*[3] but a cross reference to NHSLA advice in the area would have been useful, particularly NHSLA Circular No 02/02 *Apologies and Explanations.*[28] The circular points out the need to be careful with explanations:

> 'Care needs to be taken in the dissemination of explanations so as to avoid future litigation risks, but for the avoidance of any doubt, NHSLA will not take a point against any NHS body or any clinician seeking NHS indemnity, on the basis of a factual explanation offered in good faith before litigation is in train. We consider the provision of such information to constitute good clinical practice, and provided that facts as opposed to opinions form the basis of the explanation, nothing is likely to be revealed which would not subsequently be disclosable in the event of litigation.'

Fact and opinion: the difference?   5.26

A key point here is the difference between fact and opinion which can be difficult to distinguish in practice. Causation in clinical negligence cases is an area fraught with difficulties and an answer as to what may have caused a patient's condition may well become a legal minefield. Health staff do need to exercise extreme care in the area of explanations and apologies. Step 5 could have been developed to include something about the distinction between factual accounts and opinions.

The clinical negligence system   5.27

The organisational framework surrounding clinical risk management has been discussed. It is now necessary to consider the clinical negligence system as it shares the same NHS health quality and regulatory landscape with the organisations discussed previously in this chapter. If patient care breaks down and a patient is injured, the patient may have recourse to litigation.

Woolf   5.28

The Woolf Report[29] encapsulated all that is wrong with the clinical negligence system. Lord Woolf gave the following reasons for singling out medical negligence litigation for the most intensive examination during stage 2 of his Inquiry:

> 'The answer is that early in the Inquiry it became increasingly obvious that it was in the area of medical negligence litigation that the civil justice system was failing most conspicuously to meet the needs of litigants in a number of respects.
>
> (a) The disproportion between costs and damages in medical negligence is particularly excessive, especially in lower value cases.
>
> (b) The delay in resolving claims is more often unacceptable.
>
> (c) Unmeritorious cases are often pursued, and clear-cut claims defended, for too long.

(d)   The success rate is lower than in other personal injury litigation.

(e)   The suspicion between the parties is more intense and the lack of co-operation frequently greater than in many other areas of litigation.'

The Woolf reforms brought about judicial case management, pre-action protocols, in particular, the pre-action protocol for the resolution of clinical disputes[30] and a number of other reforms to the civil justice system. Overall views remain positive about the general thrust of the Woolf reforms.[31] The pre-action protocols seem to be working well. Experts are now less partisan and instructed in a more neutral way.

Post Woolf   5.29

Clinical negligence system reform as an issue has not stood still since the Woolf report, high profile cases of medical malpractice and damage awards have succeeded in keeping it firmly on the Government's agenda. The Kennedy Report resulting from the Bristol scandal[32] called for the review of the clinical negligence system:

> 'The system of clinical negligence litigation is now ripe for review … . The system is now out of alignment with other policy initiatives on quality and safety: in fact it serves to undermine those policies and inhibits improvements in the safety of the care received by patients.'

The report recommended the abolition of clinical negligence litigation, taking clinical error out of the courts and the tort (civil wrong) system. After the Kennedy report came the Chief Medical Officer's Call for Ideas Paper[33] followed by the consultation paper, *Making Amends*[3] which reflected both on the Woolf reforms and on the Kennedy Report as well as on some commissioned research and responses to the call for ideas.

Making Amends   5.30

The arguments for and against the present tort system were considered in *Making Amends*.[3] The idea of a comprehensive no fault system on the lines of the Swedish and New Zealand systems were considered and rejected on cost and human rights grounds. A composite package of reforms was proposed including the establishment of a NHS Redress Scheme. This scheme would have four main elements;

- an investigation of the incident;

- provision of an explanation to the patient;

- development and delivery of a package of care; and

- payments for pain and suffering etc.

Patients would be eligible for payment for serious shortcomings in NHS care if the harm could have been avoided and if causation was established. The NHS redress scheme contains a radical no-fault element proposed in relation to infant neurological impairment.Other recommendations in the report include the introduction of a duty of candour on healthcare professionals together with an exemption from disciplinary action when reporting possible negligent actions or omissions. Documents and information collected for identifying adverse events should be protected from disclosure in court.

Making Amends and the Law Society   5.31

The Law Society[34] is supportive of the basic aims of *Making Amends* but takes issue particularly with Recommendation 2, that the NHS redress scheme should encompass care and compensation for severely neurologically impaired babies, including those with severe cerebral palsy. They state that the issue of provision of care for patients and compensation for patients injured by negligence are separate ones:

> 'Children who suffer severe neurological damage as a result of negligence should receive proper compensation and we do not think that the proposed scheme is appropriate.'

They also express concern about the scope of the improvements to the provision of neurological care mentioned in this recommendation. It focuses, in their view, too narrowly and should be extended to all patients. They also see no reason why documents and information collected for identifying adverse events should be protected from disclosure in court:

> 'This will damage public confidence in the National Health Service and is contrary to the stated objectives of openness and transparency. This will give the impression to injured patients that the NHS is hiding evidence, which will be very damaging to public confidence in the system.'

Reform of the clinical negligence system   5.32

Reform of the clinical negligence system is inevitable and the only question is whether it will be a root and branch reform or whether a compromise will result accommodating the views such as those of the Law Society. *Making Amends* signals a fresh approach to clinical negligence and the report is to be broadly welcomed. The *Making Amends* proposals are radical and in principle worthy of further detailed consideration. The tort system remains but there are new structural elements introduced to help facilitate faster and perhaps more effective grievance resolution outcomes.

Conclusion   **5.33**

Clinical risk management exists in a multifarious NHS landscape of Government quangos' schemes and health policy initiatives. Surrounding all this is an adversarial focussed clinical negligence system. Together they all represent the drivers and related components of clinical risk management. The landscape of clinical risk is not an easy one to understand or negotiate. The risk manager has clearly a lot to contend with, lots of complex information to manage, understand and cascade down to others.

The concept of clinical risk management can be seen to remain very fluid. It appears as a multi-layered concept linking a number of sometimes quite disparate disciplines such as law, psychology, health policy, medicine, nursing, sociology and business management together.

As a concept it probably can never properly be clearly defined as it is too inherently diffuse by nature. It should be seen more as an intuitive concept.

Nobody really knows whether clinical risk management works or not, our best guess is that as a matter of common sense it must, we do not presently have the definitive outcome measurements to say that it definitely does. That should not however detract from us all appreciating the good efforts of all those concerned with clinical risk management and advancing health quality and patient safety.

The efforts described in this chapter and elsewhere in this book of the NHS agencies and initiatives designed to improve patient care, manage risk and improve health care dispute resolution procedures are all to be welcomed. Safe care is the pre-requisite to good quality health care.

The time must come however when the Government healthcare quality reforms stop or pause to allow NHS staff and their organisations to consolidate and reflect upon them properly. There does appear to be a constant barrage of Government initiatives in the areas discussed in this chapter and the book. The time to pause and reflect must come soon.

References

1   National Patient Safety Agency, (2003) *Seven Steps to patient safety: A guide for NHS staff*, NPSA, London.
2   Ham Chris, Dingwall Robert, Fenn Paul, Harris Don, (1988) *Medical Negligence, Compensation and Accountability*, King's Fund Institute Briefing Paper No 6, 1988, King's Fund Institute, London.
3   Department of Health, (2003) *Making Amends, A consultation paper setting out proposals for reforming the approach to clinical negligence in the NHS*, A report by the Chief Medical Officer, Department of Health, London.
4   The National Audit Office, (2001) *Handling clinical negligence claims in England*, HC 403, 3 May, The Stationery Office, London.
5   *The Health Service Ombudsman for England, Annual Report 2002–03*, HC 760, The Stationery Office, London.

6   Rosemary Bennett, 'NHS must satisfy 36 separate regulators', *The Times*, 15 October 2003.

7   Jill Sherman, 'Labour's new health quangos to be axed', *The Times*, 26 November 2003

8   NHS Reviews Coordination Group, *Improving the efficiency of scrutiny of risk management*, Progress Report, October 2003, RCG Web page www.chi.nhs.uk/nhsrcg

9   Speech by Rt Hon Alan Milburn MP, Secretary of State for Health to the New Health Network, 14 January 2002, Redefining the National Health Service, DOH, London at http://www.doh.gov.uk/speeches/jan2002milburnnhn.htm

10 Department of Health, (2001) *Shifting the Balance of Power within the NHS, Securing delivery*, Department of Health, London.

11 Lord Woolf's speech in full, *The Times*, January 17 2001, The Times On-Line, accessed 19–01–01.

12 *Doctors warn of more scandals*, BBC News Health Monday 26th June 2000, http://news.bbc.co.uk/1/hi/health/803412.stm

13 The NHS Litigation Authority, Fact sheet 1: background information, October 2003, NHSLA, London.

14 The NHS Litigation Authority, Fact sheet 3: information on claims, October 2003, NHSLA, London.

15 NHSLA Clinical Negligence Scheme for Trusts, *Clinical Risk Management Standards*, August 2003, NHSLA, London. NHSLA.

16 NHSLA, (2003) *Risk Pooling Schemes for Trusts, Risk Management Standard*, London.

17 CHI, (2002) Emerging themes from 175 clinical governance reviews, CHI, London.

18 NHSLA, *The National Health Service Litigation Authority Report and Accounts 2003*, NHSLA, London.

19 NHSLA, (2003) Clinical Negligence Scheme for Trusts, *Clinical Risk Management Standards*, London.

20 NAO, (2003) *Achieving improvements through clinical governance: A progress report on implementation by NHS trusts*, HC 1055 Session 2002–2003 17 September 2003, The Stationery Office, London.

21 *The future: CHAI-About CHAI*, Commission for Health Improvement (CHI) web page http://www.chi.nhs.uk/eng/about/chai/about.shtmlb accessed 22 January 2004.

22 CHAI, (2003) *CHAI's Vision: Purpose and Functions*, Consultative Document, Chapter 5, In the beginning, CHAI, London.

23 CHI, *An overview of clinical governance reviews*, CHI web page, www.chi.nhs.uk/eng/cgr/overview.shtml accessed 29th January 2004.

24 CHI, *Assessing clinical governance*, CHI Web page, www.chi.nhs.uk/eng/cgr/assessing.shtml accessed 4 February 2004. © 2004 Commission for Healthcare Audit and Inspection.

25 CHI, *Emerging themes from 175 clinical governance reviews*, November 2002, CHI, London.

26 Department of Health, (2000) *An organisation with a memory: Report of an expert group on learning from adverse events in the NHS*, chaired by the Chief Medical Officer, Department of Health, The Stationery Office, London.

27 Department of Health, (2001) *Building a safer NHS for patients, implementing an organisation with a memory*, , Department of Health, London.

28 NHSLA Apologies and Explanations, NHSLA Circular No02/02 11th February 2002, NHSLA, London.

29 *Access to Justice: Final Report* by The Right Honourable the Lord Woolf, Master of the Rolls, July 1996, HMSO, London.

30 Pre-action protocol for the resolution of clinical disputes, Civil Procedure Rules, Department for Constitutional Affairs, London available at www.dca.gov.uk/civil/procrules_fin/contents/protocols/prot_rcd.htm ,accessed, 3–2-04.

31 John Tingle, 'Judging the performance of the civil justice reforms', *Health Care Risk Report*, January 2003, p 10–11.

32 *Final Report, Learning from Bristol: the report of the public inquiry into children's heart surgery at the Bristol Royal Infirmary 1984–1995*, Command Paper: CM 5207, July 2001, Department of Health, London.
33 *Department of Health, (2001) Clinical negligence, what are the issues and options for reform?*, Department of Health, London.
34 The Law Society, (2003) *Making Amends, The Law Society Response*, The Law Society London.

Chapter 6
Managing Health, Safety and Environmental Risks

This chapter covers:

- The nature of health, safety and environmental risks in healthcare.

- Risk assessment.

- Legal requirements.

- HSE prosecutions in the healthcare sector.

- Corporate manslaughter and sentencing.

- Learning lessons from incidents.

- Best practice in managing health, safety and environmental risks.

- Significant health and safety risks in healthcare.

- Managing occupational health.

- Interface with clinical risk.

Introduction   6.1

The first aim of this chapter is to enhance understanding of the nature and diversity of the health, safety and environmental risks associated with healthcare delivery. The second aim is to facilitate awareness of and the ability to use effective systems to manage these risks. In addressing these two main aims a range of associated topics will be covered, including hazard and risk, risk assessment, learning lessons from past incidents and the potential consequences of failure. Some of the significant health and safety risks for the healthcare sector are covered together with the key challenges for occupational health. The interface with clinical risk issues is also explored, together with current legal and best practice requirements in relation to health, safety and environmental risks relevant to the healthcare sector.

Existing guidance   6.2

Existing guidance for the healthcare sector on health, safety and environmental risks is not in short supply. The Health and Safety Commission (HSC) through its

Health Services Advisory Committee (HSAC), and the Health and Safety Executive (HSE), have produced many documents which include general guidance on legal requirements and how to manage particular areas of risk relevant to the healthcare sector. The NHS and other organisations have also produced useful guidance. It can be confusing to successfully navigate a path through the plethora of existing guidance. The final aim of this chapter is to help to do so.

Health, safety and environmental risks in healthcare   6.3

The healthcare sector, in its broadest sense, includes hospitals (both NHS and private), ambulance services, diagnostic and research laboratories, post-mortem facilities, dental practices, GP practices, nursing and care homes, and office and teaching facilities. In a typical hospital, supporting the delivery of healthcare, are catering facilities, cleaning, building, plant and equipment maintenance, workshops, security, administrators and managers. Staff employed in the healthcare sector are therefore engaged in an extremely diverse range of work activities. Each of these work activities is associated with both common and differing health, safety and environmental risks. Some hazards present a risk not just for healthcare employees but also for patients, visitors and the environment. This can include radiation hazards, clinical waste and hazardous chemicals.

Commonly encountered risks   6.4

Individuals employed in the healthcare sector can be exposed to a broad range of risks that may result in harm. Eliminating or controlling these risks not only protects staff but is often the key to ensuring the safe and proper delivery of care. Commonly encountered risks are:

- manual handling;
- hazardous chemicals and biological agents;
- aggression and violence;
- stress; and
- ionising and non-ionising radiation.

Specific areas of risk   6.5

Particular work activities have their own attendant areas of risk. Examples include:

- **Waste disposal activities** – sharps, potentially infectious materials and manual handling risks.
- **Theatres** – anaesthetic agents, X-rays, latex, ergonomic risks, clinical waste, manual handling, infectious agents and lasers.

- **Post-mortem suites** – manual handling risks, hazardous chemicals, infectious agents, clinical waste, slips, trips and falls.

- **Diagnostic laboratories** – hazardous chemicals, flammable materials, infectious agents, equipment and electrical risks.

- **Wards** – aggression and violence, manual handling, stress, clinical waste, handling and disposal of drugs, hazardous chemicals, infectious agents, drugs, slips, trips and falls.

- **Facilities management** – construction activities, asbestos, electrical risks, hazardous chemicals, Legionella, transport, plant and equipment risks, flammable substances.

- **Administrators and managers** – stress, aggression, violence, slips, trips and falls, display screen equipment and manual handling risks.

- **Hotel service staff** – manual handling, slips, trips and falls, scalding risks, hazardous chemicals, machinery and equipment risks.

None of the above examples contain an exhaustive list of all the ways in which risk may arise, as this depends on the precise circumstances in which work is undertaken and the nature of healthcare provided. Several groups of individuals may be exposed to risk arising from a particular aspect of healthcare delivery, including staff, patients, visitors, seconded clinical and other staff, students (in teaching hospitals), and contractors.

How harm may arise   6.6

Food hygiene is an example of where there is the potential for large numbers of individuals to be exposed to harm. Food hygiene problems in hospital catering facilities have lead to outbreaks of food poisoning. Such incidents have the potential to affect staff, patients and visitors alike.

Table 6.1: Activity, risk and possible effect

Activity	Risk	Possible effect
HEALTH Anaesthesia	Inhalation of anaesthetic gases in theatres and recovery areas	Impaired behaviour and ability to work, depression of white cell formation, sensitisation of cardiac tissue, liver damage
Tissue preservation	Exposure to formaldehyde in pathology, histopathology and mortuaries	Chest tightness, coughing, occupational asthama, allergic dermatitis, sore throat, itchy eyes
Diagnostic imaging	Exposure to X-rays, ultrasound and electromagnetic fields	Cancer, hereditary defects, dermatitis

Table 6.1 (*cont'd*)

Activity	Risk	Possible effect
Invasive surgery	Exposure to body fluids and infectious agents	Hepatitis, tuberculosis, HIV, transmissible spongiform encepathology (TSE), latex allergy
SAFETY Nursing in care of the elderly	Exposure to physical and verbal abuse and manual handling	Stress, trauma, physical injury, musculoskeletal injury
Laundering of dirty linen	Exposure to cleaning agents, hazardous equipment and machinery	Skin sensitisation, physical injury, puncture wounds, scabies, hepatitis
Building and equipment maintenance	Exposure to hazardous equipment and machinery, working at heights	physical injury, electrocution and falls
ENVIRONMENT High security isolation wards	Discharge to environment of infectious organisms	Exposure of members of the public and staff to infectious disease-causing organisms
Air conditioning and ventilation for healthcare premises	Release of bacteria including legionella	Exposure of staff, patients, visitors and general public to organisms capable of causing life-threatening disease
Use of equipment containing mercury	Release or toxic chemicals from broken equipment	Exposure of staff, patients and the environment to a toxic substance during clean-up and disposal

A further example is a breakdown in infection control procedures – this can lead to widespread infection amongst patients and the staff associated with those patients. The consequences for patients who may be both susceptible to infection, for example, as a consequence of treatment with immunosuppressive drugs, and also very ill, can be extremely serious. Fatalities have resulted in the past from such incidents, and they are usually associated with a significant number of affected individuals becoming ill. Infection control problems have been magnified by the development of multi-drug resistant organisms and the consequential impact upon the successful treatment of affected individuals.

Looking in more detail at the nature of health, safety and environmental risks associated with healthcare delivery, reveals an almost bewildering array of ways in which harm may arise. Taking health, safety and the environment in turn, examples of how harm may arise are listed in **TABLE 6.1**.

Hazard and risk 6.7

Hazard and risk has been mentioned in a general risk management context in **CHAPTER 2**. Within the health and safety arena, similar definitions for hazard and risk are also used. Hazard is an intrinsic attribute of a substance or situation. It is not therefore something that can be changed or altered.

Defining hazard and risk 6.8

HSE has defined hazard in guidance on risk assessment as 'anything that can cause harm'.[1] Hazard can also be described as the potential to cause harm. Harm includes injury, ill-health, damage to plant, equipment, property and the environment, and interruption to service delivery.[2]

Risk is the probability that harm will arise. HSE has defined risk as 'the chance, high or low, that someone will be harmed by the hazard'.[2] Risk therefore depends upon the precise circumstances to which individuals are exposed, their susceptibility and the extent to which risk is controlled. Risk is therefore something that can be changed.

Determining risk exposure 6.9

An example to illustrate this is nurses working in a children's gastro-intestinal surgery ward. Following major surgery, nursing such patients is associated with the hazard of manual handling. The extent to which nursing staff are exposed will depend upon:

- the weight and height of the children;
- the extent of the patients' incapacity, or ability to move themselves;
- the availability of patient moving and handling equipment, such as slides and hoists;
- the training and encouragement of staff in the use of equipment and safe lifting techniques; and
- ward staffing levels.

In this example, the risk of injury to staff will be higher with older (and hence heavier) children, grossly incapacitated patients and where no equipment or training has been provided. Irrespective of the patient, the provision of moving and handling equipment and training in its use will reduce the risk to staff.

The difference between hazard and risk 6.10

It is important not to confuse hazard and risk. Those who make the mistake of interchanging the two terms find that this can lead to confusion in risk assessment activities. It is quite possible to have a set of work circumstances where the hazard is high but the risk of harm arising is low. There are many examples to illustrate this point. Asbestos is a good example as it has the potential to cause death (from asbestosis, lung cancer and mesothelioma) and is therefore highly hazardous; however, the risk of harm arising will be low if:

- there is negligible asbestos in the working environment;

- the asbestos-containing materials are in good condition or sealed in place so that no airborne particles arise; and

- the asbestos is inaccessible and is not scheduled to be disturbed.

Risk assessment   6.11

Once the difference between hazard and risk is understood, the process of risk assessment is straightforward. Risk assessment is the basis of health and safety legislation, whether this concerns hazardous chemicals, manual handling, display screen equipment or more general requirements to manage risk.

Steps to risk assessment   6.12

Risk assessment is a structured process that is often described in a series of steps:

- hazard identification;

- identification of who might be harmed and how;

- risk evaluation;

- documentation of risk assessment; and

- risk assessment review and revision.

Example

Imagine a loading and unloading area at the rear of a central city hospital. The area is just off a main road with heavy vehicle use. Members of the public make extensive use of a footpath alongside the loading and unloading area. The area is used for the delivery of clean linen and other hospital supplies by different subcontractors. Deliveries are normally made by lorry.

In a corner of the loading area, containers are provided for the storage of clinical waste. Hospital staff deposit clinical waste bags in these containers daily. Clinical waste is removed for disposal by specialist subcontractors by lorry. Different subcontractors also deposit cylinders of medical gases, such as oxygen, helium and anaesthetic gases, into the area. A secure compound is provided for the gas cylinders but it is too small, so full and empty cylinders are propped up against the secure compound alongside which lorries drive in and out. Hospital staff use the loading and unloading area as a short cut to reach other parts of the hospital. Illicit parking by hospital staff and visitors in the area also takes place from time to time. Loading and unloading by subcontractors is mostly unsupervised by hospital staff.

Applying the risk assessment steps in relation to this scenario would reveal the information shown in **TABLE 6.2** below.

Table 6.2: Hazard, risk and nature of risk

Hazard identification	Risk to whom	Nature of risk
Moving vehicles	Subcontractors, staff, public	Physical injury, vehicle damage, property damage
Lifting and moving heavy objects	Staff, subcontractors and staff	Musculoskeletal injuries
Falling cylinders	Staff, subcontractors, public	Physical injury
Damaged cylinders	Staff, subcontractors, public	Exposure to medical gases, physical injury, fire
Clinical waste	Staff, subcontractors, public	Fire, physical injury, infectious agents

Measures to reduce risk   6.13

The whole point of risk assessment is making decisions about whether more needs to be done to remove or control risk. Risk assessments are therefore a means to an end and not an end in themselves. Many individuals, in carrying out risk assessments, fail to go the full distance and use the information gleaned during risk assessment to identify whether further improvement is necessary.

Going the full distance with the loading and unloading example, in other words identifying what needs to be done to remove or reduce risk (risk evaluation), would reveal a number of measures that could be taken to reduce risk. These measures would include:

- the provision of a one-way system for vehicles, speed limit signs and speed bumps;
- marking out parking bays for lorries to use during loading and unloading;
- demarcated footpaths;
- signs prohibiting unauthorised access;
- security supervision of the area;
- provision of moving and lifting equipment;

- relocation of a larger cylinder store away from moving vehicles;

- prohibiting the storage of cylinders outside the cylinder store; and

- relocation of the clinical waste store so that hospital staff do not need to cross the loading and unloading area to deposit clinical waste.

Legal requirements of risk assessment   6.14

In most instances it is a legal requirement to document risk assessments. It is also good practice to do so, otherwise risk assessments will not be incorporated into day-to-day activities and may need to be unnecessarily repeated. The function of documented risk assessments is not to be filed away and dusted off in preparation for a health and safety audit, but to be an integral part of routine work activities.

It is a further legal requirement for risk assessments to be reviewed so that they remain relevant and workable. Triggers for a review include accidents or cases of ill-health, organisational change, changes to working practices and new knowledge about risk.

Health and safety legislation requires risk assessments to be suitable and sufficient. This necessitates that they address an assessment of all risks, consideration of the practicalities of preventing exposure and how risk can be removed or controlled.

Forms used in the healthcare sector for risk assessment are often overly long and complex, and require irrelevant information to be recorded. This usually leads to staff being reluctant to complete risk assessments, and therefore inadequate risk assessments. Health and safety legislation requires that risk assessments are carried out by competent individuals. Staff expected to carry out risk assessments need therefore to be trained and provided with supporting documented guidance and professional advice.

Stages of risk assessment   6.15

In order to successfully introduce risk assessment into an organisation or enhance the risk assessment process that is already in place, a sequence of stages need to be worked through. These stages include:

Risk assessment policy   6.16

- Develop a short document setting out the organisation's aspirations on risk assessment and what is to be achieved. Good policies recognise the importance of prevention of risk, substitution with less hazardous alternatives and then risk control as a hierarchical approach.

- Responsibility for completion of risk assessments, review of risk assessments and taking action to effect improvements following risk assessment, should be clearly stipulated in the policy.

- The policy should be endorsed by the chief executive or organisational head and dated.

- Circumstances which would trigger a review of the policy should also be stipulated.

Development of a risk assessment form   6.17

- Aim for an easy-to-use form, ideally on one side of A4. If IT systems allow, a computer-based form can be used.

- Seek input from health and safety professionals, occupational health, risk managers, and other staff with relevant expertise on the layout and content of the form.

- Develop clear supporting guidance which staff can easily refer to when completing the form.

- Try out the use of the form and the guidance in different parts of the organisation, seek feedback from staff and amend the form and guidance as appropriate, prior to launching throughout the organisation.

- A key part of the form is inclusion of what action is required to be taken following risk assessment, by whom and when.

Risk assessment training   6.18

- Once responsibilities have been assigned within the policy, those nominated individuals expected to complete risk assessments will need to be trained to do so. This includes doctors, nurses and other staff.

- Training can be provided in-house if individuals are available who are themselves trained and qualified to do so. Otherwise external assistance can be sought.

- All those needing to be trained should be offered a training session.

- It is important to nominate representatives from all parts of the healthcare organisation for training, also for more complex risks.

- Effective training in risk assessment can be provided by a competent trainer in a few hours.

- Training sessions should be used to emphasise the importance of the organisation's policy, to provide specific training on the use of the risk assessment form and supporting guidance.

- It is vital that training includes practical case studies.

- It is good practice to follow up training sessions with further short workshops to enable staff to raise any practical problems encountered during risk assessment. The workshops need to be scheduled a couple of months after the original training.

- Refresher and retraining courses will be needed from time to time.

Many large healthcare organisations waste time and effort on risk assessment by not harnessing the expertise of their own staff. For example, laboratory and pharmacy staff typically have much experience of completing risk assessments in relation to hazardous substances. Their expertise can be usefully deployed in developing approaches to risk assessment throughout the rest of the organisation. Such staff often have access to risk assessment forms which can be used more widely. The overall aim should be to develop a single approach to risk assessment throughout the entire organisation. The use of both different assessment forms and different approaches to assessment in different parts of the organisation is to be avoided.

Legal requirements   6.19

Within the UK, health and safety legislation has been in place for around 200 years. This legislation has the aim of protecting individuals from harm arising from work activities. The early legislation was prescriptive and addressed specific areas of risk at work, such as dangerous machinery, lead and lifting equipment. In time this was followed by legislation that dealt with particular work processes, such as construction and chemical manufacture. The piecemeal nature of the legislation continued until fairly recently when legislation reflected a more holistic and logical approach to occupational risks.

The Health and Safety at Work etc Act 1974   6.20

In 1974, ground breaking health and safety legislation was introduced, the *Health and Safety at Work etc Act 1974 (HSWA 1974)*. This Act was different from all previous health and safety legal requirements as it was not specific to particular areas of risk, work processes or sectors of employment. It addressed for the first time the process by which health and safety should be tackled within organisations 'to ensure the health, safety and welfare of employees'. In particular, the Act has specific requirements for employers to:

* provide and maintain equipment and systems of work;

* provide and maintain a safe working environment;

* prepare a health and safety policy;

* provide information, instruction, training and supervision; and

* provide adequate welfare facilities.

Crown immunity   6.21

When the Act was first introduced, although it applied to hospitals and the healthcare sector, the Crown (including the NHS), was immune from prosecution. Crown immunity was, however, lifted from the NHS in 1988, so that the full bite of these legal requirements were felt by NHS hospitals and laboratories in the same way as they were by other sectors of employment. This late move of all of the healthcare sector under the umbrella of health and safety legal requirements, in comparison to other sectors of employment, was one of the reasons behind comparatively poor standards of health and safety in hospitals and other healthcare establishments at that time.

HSE powers 6.22

Health and safety legislation that applies to workplace activities, including the provision of healthcare, is criminal law. The legislation is enforced in healthcare premises (such as hospitals, care homes, GP surgeries, dental surgeries, health centres and clinics) by HSE inspectors. HSE inspectors have far-reaching powers which include:

- access to work premises at any reasonable time;

- freedom to interview staff, contractors, visitors and patients;

- taking of statements, photographs, measurements and samples;

- confiscation of equipment and documents;

- issue of notices (Improvement and Prohibition) requiring, respectively, improvements by a certain date or stopping a work activity until improvements are made; and

- initiation of criminal court proceedings for alleged breaches of health and safety legislation.

Where cases are heard 6.23

Most cases involving contravention of health and safety legislation are heard in the magistrates' courts. Such cases are either heard by a district judge or a bench of two or three lay magistrates. The maximum penalties that can be imposed by the magistrates' courts varies according to the legislation involved; at the moment they range from £5,000–£20,000 or six months' imprisonment.

Crown Court cases 6.24

Cases involving a more serious set of circumstances, such as a fatality or serious injury or a more serious breach of the legislation, may be referred to a Crown Court for hearing. The significance of this for defendants is that, if convicted, there is no limit to the penalty that a Crown Court can impose. In theory, therefore, higher fines may result in comparison to those set by the magistrates; in practice, however, this is not always the case. Cases involving breaches of health and safety legislation are known as triable either way – that is, both the prosecutor (HSE) and the defendant (the healthcare organisation or individual) can elect for trial in a Crown Court. In the past the prosecutor usually chose the venue, although some defendants selected a Crown Court as the venue, believing that a fairer verdict would be delivered by a jury.

In consequence of recent changes, defendants are now required to enter a plea (guilty or not guilty) and the courts then decide on the appropriate venue for the hearing. It is not unusual for Crown Court cases, particularly if they are defended, to last for several days or weeks. The associated legal costs can therefore be significant, but perhaps worth the risk to a defendant who truly believes they are innocent. It should, however, be borne in mind that HSE has an impressive track record in securing convictions for breaches of legislation. Defendants should therefore not make decisions lightly to defend the case or for the case to be heard in a Crown Court.

Defendants in HSE prosecutions   6.25

In most instances cases will be brought against the employing organisation, such as an NHS trust. A number of trusts have recently been successfully prosecuted by HSE for breaches of health and safety legislation. A summary of some of these cases appears in **6.26–6.32 BELOW** Prior to the creation of trusts, health authorities were also successfully prosecuted. The reason that most cases are brought against the employing organisation is that health and safety legislation confers extensive duties on employers. Investigation by HSE inspectors of either a workplace incident or during a routine visit or audit invariably identifies failures by the employer to meet legal requirements. A number of HSE prosecutions have, however, been taken against individuals, such as those engaged in running nursing and care homes.

HSE prosecutions in the healthcare sector   6.26

The following are examples of prosecutions that HSE have successfully persued in the healthcare sector. They are interesting examples of the circumstances that can give rise to court cases and demonstrate that compliance with legal duties in relation to employees is just as relevant as ensuring that others (patients and visitors to healthcare premises) are not exposed to risk.

Collapsed balcony   6.27

In April 2000, a young man fell from a balcony and died from his injuries. The balcony was on the second floor of a residential block for student nurses belonging to a NHS trust. The balcony was an architectural feature rather than a true balcony on which people could stand. Prior to the incident the deceased had been drinking and witnesses saw him on the balcony. The balcony was poorly maintained and described in court as being in 'a dilapidated condition'. The deceased may have interferred with the balcony railings and hence may have contributed to the subsequent collapse of the balcony, although this was not conclusively proved.

HSE prosecuted the NHS trust alleging that it had failed to comply with *section 3* of the *HSWA 1974* which requires: '… every employer to conduct his undertaking in such a way as to ensure, so far as is reasonably practicable, that persons not in his employment who may be affected thereby are not thereby exposed to risks to their health or safety.' The trust entered a not guilty plea to the charge but were found guilty by the Court in 2002. The district judge concluded that the condition of the balcony was such that it exposed a person on it to risk to his health and safety. The judge was further of the view that it was reasonably practicable for the trust to have taken steps to prevent the risk as the balcony could have been repaired, or the window leading to the balcony could have been fitted with a bar to prevent access to the balcony. As the trust took neither of these steps they had therefore failed to comply with *HSWA 1974*.

Cardiac angiography 6.28

This case demonstrates the application of health and safety legal requirements to clinical procedures, a fact which is frequently over-looked by healthcare managers and clinicians. The case was the first to be taken by HSE in relation to the death of a patient undergoing clinical procedures. The case concerns cardiac angiography, a diagnostic imaging procedure in which contrast medium is introduced by injection into the blood vessels supplying the heart. Unfortunately the procedure was not carried out correctly and rather than contrast medium, air was injected into the patient resulting in a fatal air embolism.

There were three members of the trust's staff engaged in the procedure – a radiographer under training, a second radiographer and a cardiologist. The former fitted an empty syringe into the equipment's pump mechanism prior to the end of the morning session. After lunch, the second radiographer attended but did not check whether the syringe had been filled with contrast medium. The cardiologist thought he saw contrast medium coming from the free end of the syringe tubing and proceeded to connect it to the catheter to the patient's heart.

The subsequent investigation was jointly conducted by HSE and the Medical Devices Agency (MDA). The MDA concluded that the equipment was not faulty. HSE were concerned about the lack of procedures for the safe hand-over of the equipment (a safe system of work), and concluded that the trust had failed to meet the requirements of *section 3* of the *HSWA 1974*. The trust pleaded guilty and the case was heard in the Magistrates' Court but referred to the Crown Court for sentencing. The Magistrates did this in order that a higher penalty could be considered, as they felt the maximum fine they could impose was inadequate. The Crown Court imposed a fine of £38,000 and the trust had additionally to meet the prosecution's costs of £17,000. The sentencing judge was of the view that:

' … a health service trust is responsible for having in being a reasonable safe system of work, even though the service which it operates involves the services of experts … . The purpose of the law in this field is to ensure that the employer does not rest upon the assumptions that those he employs will always do the obvious.'

HSE inspection   6.29

In August 1997, a NHS trust was prosecuted following an inspection carried out
by HSE of one of its hospitals. During the inspection a wide range of poor health
and safety practices were encountered which lead HSE to conclude that this was
evidence of a more fundamental managerial failing within the trust.[3]

During the inspection, a catalogue of problems were identified including:

- inadequate arrangements for handling clinical waste;
- poor arrangements for manual handling;
- unsafe practices during post-mortems;
- inappropriate sharps procedures; and
- poor electrical safety.

Within the laboratory used for processing suspect tuberculosis specimens, the
facilities were such that HSE issued a Prohibition Notice which prevented the
laboratory from being used until certain improvements had been made.

Risk management consultants had previously advised the trust to appoint a health
and safety adviser. The trust's Risk Management Committee decided that priority
ought to be directed to other areas of risk that the trust faced at that time, such as
fire precautions and clinical risk. The trust was engaged in one of the first healthcare PFI projects to build a new hospital and this is likely to have consumed
senior management time and energy. The trust had however failed to realise that
compliance with health and safety legal requirements is not something that can be
periodically addressed, it is a continual and ever present requirement.

The case was heard in a Magistrates' Court and concerned a failure to comply
with *regulation 4* of the *Management of Health and Safety at Work Regulations 1992
(SI 1992/2051)*. Regulation 4 relates to effective planning, organisation, control,
monitoring and review. The trust was fined £4,000 of a maximum fine of
£5,000 and ordered to pay the prosecution's costs.

This case is interesting for a number of reasons. Firstly the case did not follow on
from an accident in which someone was harmed. Secondly the health and safety
arrangements within the trust were not entirely flawed as good documented policies existed, managers were committed to health and safety and staff co-operated
to resolve health and safety issues. Thirdly the case demonstrated that diligent
middle managers are not sufficient in the absence of a more senior and corporate
demonstrable commitment to health and safety. The Chief Executive of the trust
tendered his resignation which was accepted a few days after the court case.

Deaths during anaesthesia   6.30

Two cases were taken by HSE in relation to two patient fatalities which occurred
in 2000 and 2002. The circumstances of the incidents were similar and related to

elderly patients admitted for surgery to a University Hospital who were undergoing anaesthesia. Contrary to the manufacturer's instructions a peep valve was permanently connected to the anaesthetic machine. The valve was around five years old at the time of the second patient fatality and had not been maintained in that time. The valve was examined by the MDA and found to be heavily corroded – an indication of the absence of maintenance. Whilst the patients were being anaesthetised, the peep valve actuated which resulted in the patients not being able to exhale. In both instances the patients died.

HSE, at the conclusion of their joint investigation with the MDA, instituted legal proceedings against the trust. The trust was accused of failing to comply with *section 3* of the *HSWA 1974* in relation to their responsibilities towards the two patients. Two separate cases under *section 3* of the *HSWA 1974* were taken in relation to the patient deaths. At the subsequent court hearing, in which the trust pleaded guilty to both charges, a fine of £15,000 was imposed in relation to the second death and a further fine of £12,000 in relation to the first incident. The trust also paid HSE's costs of £2,400.

These cases illustrate some serious failures in the trust who allowed the circumstances which gave rise to the death of the first patient to persist for several years until the second patient died. This clearly demonstrates an absence of learning from a prior and very serious event. These cases were heard in the Magistrates Court. Given the severity of the outcome of the incidents and the fact that the unsafe situation existed for such a long period of time, the trust was fortunate that the cases were not referred to the Crown Court for sentencing, where heavier penalties could well have been imposed.

Exposure to a hazardous chemical 6.31

Two trust employees were in the process of carrying out work on PVC pipe work in connection with a swimming pool. The work was undertaken in an enclosed duct below the pool. The repair work involved the use of a hazardous chemical, methyl ethyl ketone (MEK). The duct was a confined space with limited ventilation. A preliminary risk assessment had recognised the problem of ventilation and indicated that a fan should be used for work in the duct. Whilst the repair work was undertaken the pool was in use and so a decision was made to keep a hatch to the duct closed. Although the fan was used in the duct, the hatch was shut and so ventilation remained inadequate. As the repair work got underway, the employees accidentally spilt the MEK in the duct. One of the employees was overcome by the chemical fumes and collapsed in the duct. He was pulled free of the duct by a colleague.

An investigation of the incident revealed a number of problems:

● a proper risk assessment for the repair work had not been carried out;

● the risk of working in confined spaces had not been fully appreciated nor indeed what actually constituted a confined space;

- the employees had not been properly trained in confined space work nor the circumstances under which MEK should not be used; and

- there were no rescue procedures in place for confined space work.

The trust was prosecuted by HSE for failing to comply with the *HSWA 1974*, *Management of Health and Safety at Work Regulations 1999 (SI 1999/3242)*, *Confined Spaces Regulations 1997 (SI 1997/1713)* and *Control of Substances Hazardous to Health Regulations 2002 (SI 2002/2677) (COSHH Regulations 2000)*. The court imposed a total fine of £7,000 on the trust. The trust had additionally to pay HSE costs of just over £2,000.

Patient suicide   6.32

In January 2004, the headline in the local newspaper read 'Trust fined £10,000.00 after patient suicide'.[6] This was a Scottish case heard in the Sheriff Court and concerned the suicide of a mentally ill patient in a PCT. The patient had been allocated to a single room in the hospital's acute admissions/secure unit. The deceased had suffered a depressive illness for around four years prior to admission. In the days immediately prior to her death staff had heard the patient say she 'wanted to go to a better place' and she 'wished to be dead'. She had also broken windows in her room either in preparation for escape or to injure herself. On the day prior to her death constant observation was ceased as her frame of mind was thought to have improved. On the evening of the next day, the patient was found in her room by a member of staff. The patient had hung herself from a window fixing known as an eyelet. Despite emergency assistance the patient died.

Seven months prior to this incident, HSE had investigated the circumstances of an attempted suicide in the same ward of the hospital. The circumstances were very similar in that a patient had attempted to hang himself from a window eyelet. Internal memos indicated the urgency of removing the window fixings following the attempted suicide, but the work was not carried out, despite the clear indication of the risk involved.

The trust pleaded guilty to the charge of failing to comply with *section 3* of the *HSWA 1974* in relation to psychiatric patients. The Sheriff hearing the case commented:

> 'We have seen that ... the risk posed to patients using such a window eyelet to commit suicide had been graphically illustrated. The risk was recognized and it was recommended that alternative window catches be considered as a matter of urgency. Had that been done we would not have been faced with the suicide of ... . This is a serious matter that, of course, had serious and tragic consequences'.

The case was the first of its type to be heard in Scotland and will have significant ramifications for trusts and other bodies engaged in the provision of care to patients at risk of suicide. Again the circumstances demonstrate the serious consequences of failing to learn from incidents and implement improvements to prevent further risk arising.

Corporate manslaughter   6.33

There remains active consideration of amending health and safety law to cover corporate manslaughter more properly. One of the drivers for this is the number of major incidents over the years involving multiple fatalities of members of the public or employees. Such incidents include:

* the 1987 Zeebrugge ferry disaster, 189 deaths;

* the 1987 King's Cross fire, 31 deaths;

* the 1988 Clapham Rail crash, 35 deaths and 500 injured;

* the 1988 Piper Alpha fire and explosion, 167 deaths; and

* the 1999 Paddington rail crash, seven deaths and 151 injured.

Investigation of these incidents has revealed a catalogue of corporate and individual failures.

The Paddington rail crash case   6.34

Following the Paddington rail crash, the train driver was indicted for seven manslaughter charges and a further case was brought against him for failing to discharge his duties as an employee under *section 7 of HSWA 1974*. Great Western Trains were indicted for seven counts of corporate manslaughter and for failing to comply with *HSWA 1974, s 3*. In the Paddington rail crash a high speed train travelling from Swansea to London passed a red signal (a signal passed at danger or SPAD) which led to the train colliding with a freight train. At the time of the collision, the onboard safety system was inoperative.

In court (*R v Great Western Trains [1999] Unreported*), legal arguments centred around the negligence of individuals and determining the directing mind in an organisation. The judge hearing the case stated: 'It is still necessary to look for such a directing mind and identify where gross negligence is that fixes the company with criminal responsibility.'[5]

Calls for stronger legislation   6.35

This case, as have others before it, such as *R v P&O European Ferries (Dover) Ltd [1991] 93 Cr. App R72* following the Zeebrugge ferry disaster, demonstrated the difficulty of securing corporate manslaughter convictions under existing legislation. This has led to calls for the existing legislation to be strengthened to enable more appropriate legal proceedings to be instituted.

A 1996 Law Commission report (*Involuntary manslaughter: Law Commission report 237*, Law Commission, London) recommended new legislation and a draft bill was prepared, to create new offences of reckless killing by gross carelessness and corporate killing, to replace the offence of manslaughter in cases where death is caused without the intention of causing death or serious injury.

Proposals for changing the law 6.36

In May 2001, the then Home Secretary, Jack Straw, announced a consultation document on involuntary manslaughter and proposals for changing existing legislation. The proposals largely followed the earlier Law Commission recommendations but contained some significant differences. The proposals stated that a corporation would be guilty of corporate killing if:

(a)   a management failure by the corporation is the cause or one of the causes of a person's death; and

(b)   that failure constitutes conduct falling far below what can reasonably be expected in the circumstances.

If a corporate body is found guilty, it is proposed they will be liable to an unlimited fine. It is worth noting at this point the penalties that have been imposed in a number of recent cases where organisations and individuals were found guilty of breaches of health, safety and environment legislation.

If corporate manslaughter legislation is tightened up, is it is a matter for debate and courtroom experience whether the legislation will have the desired impact – that is, to hold corporate bodies legally liable for serious accidents. Proposals for this legislative change were not however included in the last Queen's speech in 2003.

Recent penalties for breaches 6.37

- In 1999, London Underground Ltd was fined £300,000 for breaches of *section 3* of the *HSWA 1974* and the *Management of Health and Safety at Work Regulations 1992 (SI 1992/2051)*. The cases followed an accident where a passenger fell between the train and the platform at a Piccadilly line station.

- Following the Heathrow Airport tunnel collapse in 1999, Balfour Beatty was fined £1.2 million.

- The Environmental Agency secured a fine of £4 million against Millford Haven Port Authority following the leak of 72,000 tonnes of oil from the 'Sea Express'. The case was brought under the *Water Resources Act 1991*. Following appeal by the defendants, the fine was reduced to £75,000.

- In 2000, following an accident to an employee who was fatally injured when transferring waste into a tip, the owner of the company was sentenced to twelve months' imprisonment and suspended for two years.

Death in relation to a work activity 6.38

Where death occurs in relation to a work activity, investigation into the circumstances is normally undertaken by the health and safety enforcing authority (HSE in the case of healthcare organisations) and the police. The focus of a police investigation is to establish whether the circumstances constitute manslaughter. The focus of an HSE investigation is to establish whether health and safety legislation has been complied with.

There have been several cases of manslaughter that have been tried in relation to patient fatalities. Cases of manslaughter have been instituted against healthcare employees, including consultants, where patients have died as a consequence of a medication error. These errors have arisen either due to alleged gross negligence on the part of the staff involved or due to intentional harm.

Breaches of professional duty of care where there is recklessness or gross negligence may also constitute manslaughter. *R v Adomako [1994] 4 All ER 935* a leading case on this concerns an anaesthetist who during surgery failed to notice that the oxygen tube to the patient from a ventilator became disconnected. The patient suffered a cardiac arrest and subsequently died. The defendant anaesthetist was charged with involuntary manslaughter and convicted on the basis that he had been grossly negligent and there had been a gross dereliction of care.

More recently the outbreak of Legionnaires' Disease in Barrow in Furness, has resulted in a local authority middle manager being charged with manslaughter. The outbreak lead to the death of several members of the public. This case illustrates the importance of managers acting responsibly and carefully to ensure that individuals are not exposed to risk.

The increase in workplace fatalities over recent years is a further driver for corporate manslaughter. HSE figures for 2000/01 show a 34% increase in fatalities in comparison with the previous year. There are many, not just trade unions, who feel that the introduction of corporate manslaughter legislation is the most appropriate way to tackle this unacceptable tide of workplace deaths. It is, however, important to point out that under current plans it will not impact upon death caused by chronic exposure to, for example, hazardous chemicals or chronic injury from manual handling.

Sentencing   6.39

The leading case that is used for guiding sentencing of offences under health, safety and environment legislation is *R v F Howe & Sons (Engineering) Ltd [1999] 2 All ER 249*. This Court of Appeal case concerned a fatal accident to an employee of the company who was electrocuted whilst cleaning the appellant's factory with an electric vacuum cleaner. The cleaner was used to suck up water from the factory floor. The company had therefore failed to ensure the health and safety at work of one of its employees and 'the lack of a system to check its electrical equipment fell far short of the appropriate standard'.

The judge hearing the appeal stated that penalties should be determined on a case by case basis. From that case, aggravating and mitigating factors which are now taken into consideration by the criminal courts in determining penalty include:

- Aggravating factors:
    - a failure to heed warnings;
    - whether a death has occurred; and
    - whether a deliberate breach of health and safety legislation has taken place with a view to maximising profit.
- Mitigating factors:
    - prompt admission of responsibility;
    - an early plea of guilty;
    - steps implemented to remedy deficiences and prevent a recurrence; and
    - an otherwise good health and safety performance.

It is expected that before trial, the prosecution and defence will agree on the aggravating and mitigating factors. This follows on from the case *R v Friskies Pet Care Co [2000] 2 Cr App R(S) 401* in 2000 where the court adopted the practice of the prosecution serving a list of aggravating factors and the defendant responding with a list of mitigating factors. However, where there is an offence under the *HSWA 1974* which has lead to death or serious injury, then in line with the judgement in the Howe case, such cases will be referred to the Crown Court.

Whilst the maximum penalties that a court can impose are established, in practice the overriding criterion in establishing penalty is ability to pay. In consequence, courts often have difficulty in setting fines where the defendant is from the public sector, and can be swayed by the lack of financial reserves in NHS healthcare providers. In the case of *R v Milford Haven Port Authority [2000] 2 Cr App Rep (S) 423*, the judge stated that if a substantial financial penalty will inhibit a public body from discharging its function then this should be taken into account in setting the fine.

Main legislation 6.40

The main health and safety legislation in the UK remains the *Health and Safety at Work etc Act 1974*. This legislation forms the basis for all other occupational health and safety legislation.

Examples of health, safety and environmental legislation relating to the healthcare sector

Health and Safety at Work etc Act 1974

Management of Health and Safety at Work Regulations 1999 (SI 1999/3242)

Control of Substances Hazardous to Health Regulations 2002 (SI 2002/2677) (COSHH)

Manual Handling Operations Regulations 1992 (SI 1992/2793)

Display Screen Equipment Regulations 1992 (SI 1992/2792)

Personal Protective Equipment Regulations 1992 (SI 1992/2966)

Ionising Radiation Regulations 1999 (SI 1999/3232)

Electricity at Work Regulations 1989 (SI 1989/635)

Noise at Work Regulations 1989 (SI 1989/1790)

Genetically Modified Organisms (Contained Use) Regulations 1992 (SI 1992/3217)

Genetically Modified Organisms (Contained Use) (Amendment) Regulations 1996 (SI 1996/967)

Health and Safety (First-Aid) Regulations 1981 SI 1981/917)

Health and Safety (Consultation with Employees) Regulations 1996 (SI 1996/1513)

Safety Representatives and Safety Committess Regulations 1977 (SI 1977/500)

Reporting of Injuries, Diseases and Dangerous Occurences Regulations 1995 (SI 1995/3163) (RIDDOR)

Working Time Regulations 1998 (SI 1998/1933)

Provision and Use of Work Equipment Regulations 1998 (SI 1998/2306)

Lifting Operations and Lifting Equipment Regulations 1998 (SI 1998/2307)

Health and Safety (Miscellaneous Amendments) Regulations 2002 (SI 2002/2174)

Workplace (Health, Safety and Welfare) Regulations 1992 (SI 1992/3004)

Construction (Design and Management) Regulations 1994 (SI 1994/3140)

Construction (Health Safety and Welfare) Regulations 1996 (SI 1996/1592)

Control of Asbestos at Work Regulations 2002 (SI 2002/2675)

Asbestos (Licensing) Regulations 1983 (SI 1983/1649)

Dangerous Substances and Explosive Atmospheres Regulations 2002 (SI 2002/2776)

Environmental Protection Act 1990

The *HSWA 1974* specifies the general duties of employers towards employees and others, which includes members of the public and patients in the context of healthcare delivery. It also specifies the duties of employees to themselves and each other.

Reasonable practicability   6.41

The duties are qualified by the clause 'so far as is reasonably practicable'. Reasonable practicability entails a balanced decision and that decision is based upon risk assessment. Reasonably practicable therefore depends upon:

● the degree of risk; and

● the time, trouble, cost and difficulty involved in removing or controlling risk.

The amount of time, trouble and cost expended should not be grossly dispropor-tionate to the risk. In demonstrating to HSE inspectors and proving to the crimi-nal courts that reasonably practicable steps have been taken, clearly the greater the risk the more will be expected to be done to remove or control it. In meeting the test of reasonably practicable the principles of sound management and common sense need to be kept to the fore.

Management Regulations   6.42

In 1992, the implicit requirements of the *HSWA 1974* to manage risk were made somewhat more explicit by the introduction of the *Management of Health and Safety at Work Regulations 1992 (SI 1992/2051)*. These Regulations, usually referred to as the 'Management Regulations' were updated in 1999. Like the *HSWA 1974*, the Management Regulations apply to all work activities. A key part of the Regulations is a general requirement for risk assessment. Prior to these Regulations, the requirement for risk assessment was confined to legislation deal-ing with particular risks, such as hazardous substances, lead and asbestos. Further requirements under the Management Regulations relate to:

● making arrangements to implement health and safety measures;

● appointment of competent advisers;

● establishment of emergency procedures;

● provision of information and training; and

● cooperation with other employers sharing the same workplace.

The later requirement is particularly pertinent to healthcare organisations, where, for example, in large hospitals, employees of the trust may work alongside univer-sity staff, out-sourced professional services, (such as occupational health) and Health Protection Agency staff. *Regulation 21* of the *Management Regulations 1999 (SI 1999/3242)* contains a significant change as employers can no longer use an act or default caused by an employee or a competent person as a defence.

The consequences of failing to manage risks   6.43

The impact upon organisations and individuals of failing to manage health, safety and environmental risks can be very significant. The impact can include all or some of the following:

For organisations (employers):

- tarnished reputation;

- loss of contracts;

- delayed service delivery;

- loss of key staff;

- unplanned managerial time spent reacting to incidents;

- court fines;

- legal costs;

- compensation claims;

- high staff turnover; and

- increased insurance premiums.

For individuals (employees):

- reduced capacity for work;

- redeployment;

- retraining;

- reduced earning capacity;

- early retirement;

- death;

- disability;

- reduced quality of life;

- loss of valued work colleagues; and

- imprisonment.

The emotional impact   6.44

These lists, however, give little indication of the emotional impact of serious workplace failures to manage risk. No one expects their partner, family member, work colleague or friend to not come home at the end of the working day because they have been killed or seriously injured in a workplace incident. Whilst the percentage of the annual total of employee fatalities which occur in the healthcare sector is small in comparison with, for example, the construction sector, each fatality or serious injury is one too many. A recent fatal accident in a hospital illustrates the impact of workplace incidents (see box below).

Death by asphyxiation

In 1999, a research council employee working at a hospital died of asphyxiation. The individual had been filling containers with liquid nitrogen. He was already dead when he was found on the floor of the liquid nitrogen room by a colleague. This second employee fell in the room and struck her head whilst shutting off a liquid nitrogen bulk supply tank. She and her deceased colleague were subsequently dragged from the room by her supervisor. A total of five employees were admitted to hospital. It is not difficult to imagine that more than one member of staff could have died in this incident.

How the incident happened

The incident arose because of an unsafe system of work which was used during the liquid nitrogen filling process. A number of factors contributed to the depleted levels of oxygen in the filling room, including:

- inadequate extract ventilation to clear nitrogen from the room;

- inadequate arrangements to allow for fresh air to enter the room;

- inactivation of the oxygen alarm warning of low oxygen levels;

- a leak in the liquid nitrogen storage tank allowing nitrogen to leak into the filling room; and

- lack of awareness amongst staff using the room as to the purpose of the oxygen alarm.

HSE investigation

The HSE investigation of this incident concluded that several requirements of both the *HSWA 1974* and the *Management Regulations* had not been complied with. The employer was prosecuted by HSE and fined £25,000.

Learning lessons from incidents   6.45

CHAPTER 4 has addressed the importance of using incidents as learning opportunities. All incidents, whether involving actual harm or the potential for harm to arise, present opportunities to learn what went wrong and what needs to be done so that the incident does not arise again. This is as relevant in the management of health, safety and environmental risks as it is in other areas of risk management. Amongst health and safety professionals this is well-trodden ground as they have long used incidents in this way. It is worthwhile, therefore, looking at the specific impact on health, safety and environmental risks that incidents may present.

The Piper Alpha tragedy   6.46

In relatively recent years one of the most major workplace incidents was the Piper Alpha tragedy in 1988. Following a major explosion and fire on the offshore platform, 167 workers lost their lives. A formal inquiry was held into the disaster in order to establish what had led to the incident. The inquiry uncovered a number of technical and organisational failures. In keeping with incidents in general, whether major or minor, a series of failures had occurred which led up to the disaster; rarely do incidents involve a single isolated failure.

The Piper Alpha inquiry identified error in maintenance procedures which eventually led to the leak which gave rise to the explosion and fire. The maintenance errors were attributed to inexperienced workers, poor maintenance procedures and poor organisational learning. There was a breakdown of communication on the platform and also to a sister platform which contributed to the scale of the incident. There was further breakdown in the permit-to-work system during shift changeover and safety procedures were insufficiently practised. The inquiry also revealed a number of human factor issues associated with the behaviour of individuals during emergency evacuation procedures and the ability of those in charge of the platform to retain authoritative control during a major disaster.

The accident pyramid   6.47

Piper Alpha was a complex disaster involving a series of failures which contributed to the precise nature of the incident and the devastating outcome. Major disasters such as this are, however, 'top-tier' events in an accident pyramid. Top-tier events do not occur every day whereas more minor incidents and near-misses can be commonplace. The important point is that the underlying root causes of minor incidents and major disasters can be the same. Chance plays its part in a series of failures coinciding and hence the final outcome. Risk management can do nothing to influence chance but it can identify and rule out failures and in so doing reduce the numbers of incidents which arise and the severity of their outcome.

Similar patterns of failure   6.48

Investigation of incidents arising within healthcare often reveal similar patterns of failure. Typically these include:

●   a breakdown in communication;

●   an absence of training;

●   lack of risk assessment;

- lack of documented policy or guidance;

- lack of resources;

- conflicting demands placed on staff;

- no monitoring of working practice; and

- lack of commitment to managing risk at the top of the organisation.

The incident described earlier in which a research worker was asphyxiated illustrates a number of these failures. If there was a risk assessment for the nitrogen filling process, clearly it was not adequate. Staff were not trained in alarm and evacuation procedures. A further failure was in the provision of extraction and make-up air.

Learning opportunities   6.49

The learning opportunities from minor incidents or near-misses which do not result in harm should not be overlooked; they will be more numerous and if circumstances were different they could give rise to harm. Near-misses may also be more easy to investigate, as staff will be less concerned about their individual culpability.

Key lessons can be learnt about day-to-day working practices when incident information is combined with claims and complaints. A ward or department with a significant claims, complaints and incident history may be indicative of a fundamental management problem dependent upon the precise background, whereas an area of the organisation which has few complaints, a small number of minor unrepeated incidents and is associated with a high level of patient thank-you letters is likely to be in a different league in effective risk management.

Best practice in managing risks   6.50

Legislation contains minimal requirements for managing health, safety and environmental risks. Whilst compliance with legal requirements normally goes hand in hand with significant reduction in the numbers of workplace accidents,[6] any further improvement in performance entails going beyond legal requirements.

Many sectors of employment have developed their own specific responses to ensuring best practice in health, safety and environmental management. Such developments are often led by industry associations and other representative bodies, such as the Confederation of British Industry and the Chemical Industries Association. The healthcare sector is perhaps less fortunate than other sectors in that it does not have such long established representative bodies acting as the focus for the development of best practice. There is, however, nothing to stop risk management professionals in healthcare from looking at initiatives in other sectors to enhance performance and benchmarking in their own sector.

There is increasing evidence to indicate that these professionals are forming representative groups to take forward initiatives in the healthcare sector. Professional bodies IOSH and BOSH (Institution of Occupational Safety and Health and the British Occupational Hygiene Society respectively), both have specialist healthcare groups, facilitating networking amongst risk professionals and the sharing of experience.

Guidance available   6.51

There are numerous documented approaches available which can guide best practice in managing health, safety and environmental risks in healthcare. Unlike other sectors these approaches are less coordinated, so it is necessary to look in many directions to resolve the best way forward. Currently it is important to consider the following:

- controls assurance standards and supporting guidance;

- guidance from HSC's Health Services Advisory Committee (HSAC);

- NHSE guidelines on health and safety issues;

- HSE guidance *Successful Health and Safety Management*;

- British Standard Institute guidance on health and safety management;

- Guidance from the Department of Health, Medical Devices Agency (MDA), Medicines Control Agency (and their successor organisation the Medicines and Healthcare Products Regulation Agency (MHRA)), Advisory Committee on Dangerous Pathogens (ACDP) and Advisory Committee on Genetic Modication (ACGM) on health, safety and environmental issues associated with healthcare;

- HSC Approved Codes of Practice on specific legal requirements; and

- CHAI guidance.

A route map through the guidance   6.52

A suggested route map through this plethora of best practice guidance is as follows:

- Legal requirements are not optional and as HSE, HSAC, ACDP, ACGM guidance is closely linked to legal duties and specific healthcare risks, start with these, and in particular the Approved Codes of Practice which have been developed in association with specific legislation and set out the route to compliance.

- HSE's *Successful Health and Safety Management*[2] is a crucial document to use in the development of approaches to best practice, so move onto this next.

- Then move on to the closely related HSAC guidance on Management of Health and Safety in the Health Services[7], as this translates the previous HSE guidance for the healthcare sector.

147

- If general help is still needed on developing best practice approaches, consider the British Standard, but in real terms this adds little to the HSE and HSAC guidance.

- Once a general approach has been developed, supplement this with approaches to managing specific areas of risk by using HSE, DoH, MDA, ACDP and ACGM guidance as appropriate.

New developments   6.53

Keeping up to speed on new developments in best practice is a task that needs to be undertaken on a routine basis. One of the easiest ways to do this is by searching the websites of relevant organisations. A number of commercial organisations also produce CD-ROM and software-based information which is regularly updated with new legal and best practice requirements. Some of these incorporate particularly useful word searches to help identify key guidance from all the main organisations. It is, however, important to understand the relative hierarchy of all the best practice guidance in order to develop a meaningful approach that does not involve wasted effort.

Keeping up with government thinking   6.54

In 1999, deputy prime minister John Prescott announced an initiative with a number of aims in the health and safety arena. He proposed:

- a strategic appraisal of the health and safety framework;

- a new agenda for the first 25 years of the new millennium; and

- reducing the impact of health and safety failures by 30% over ten years.

This was followed in June 2000 by the launch of *Revitalising Health and Safety*.[8] The background to this document was a deeply held concern for the number of deaths in the workplace and the associated societal costs, which were estimated to be £18 billion per year.

Targets   6.55

One part of best practice in managing health, safety and environmental risks is therefore currently to comply with the targets set in the *Revitalising* document. Unlike other sectors, these targets are not generally uppermost in the minds of healthcare managers and risk management specialists. They are nevertheless key targets to work towards. Targets for Great Britain have been set by the Government to:

- reduce working days lost per 100,000 workers from work-related injury and ill-health by 30% by 2010;

- reduce incidence rate of fatal and major injuries by 10% by 2010;

- reduce incidence rate of work-related ill-health by 20% by 2010; and

- achieve half the above by 2004.

These targets lend further importance to the need to have effective incident recording systems and analytical arrangements in place. Without such systems it is impossible to set targets and know when they have been achieved. In organisations where there is no maturity in incident recording systems, as is the case for many healthcare providers, the introduction of targets for accident reduction can be counter-productive and merely drive down reporting levels. Thorough planning and careful communication within the organisation is therefore necessary if this particular aspect of best practice is to succeed.

Further motivations for achievement of best practice are currently being considered by the Government. These include:

- linking court penalties for breaches of health and safety legislation to turnover or profit;

- prohibition of directors' bonuses for a fixed period;

- suspension of managers without pay; and

- suspended sentences pending remedial action.

In July 2000, HSE produced *Securing Health Together*[9] which set out its occupational health strategy for England, Scotland and Wales. The strategy adds detail on occupational health targets following the earlier *Revitalising* document. Specific targets for achievement by 2010 are:

- a 20% reduction on the incidence of work-related ill-health;

- a 20% reduction in ill-health to members of the public caused by a work activity; and

- a 30% reduction in the number of working days lost due to work-related ill-health.

Whilst targets, particularly in the long neglected area of occupational health, are important, many organisations will find these distinctly 'un-SMART'. Most organisations, including those in the healthcare sector, have no accurate data on occupational ill-health and the second target is particularly challenging for the sector, where patients die whether despite best efforts or because of a failure in care. Cynicism apart, these HSE targets should be viewed as a spur to improving the health at work of employees and ensuring that arrangements are in place to prevent exposure to risks to health.

Using available expertise   6.56

One key part of securing best practice concerns the use that is made within organisations of available expertise. Most large organisations, including those in the healthcare sector, have access to in–house risk management expertise. Rarely is it the case, however, that the in–house health and safety and occupational health provision expertise is deployed to maximum effect. In order for best practice to be achieved such expertise needs to be given the credibility that it deserves. All too often, however, these risk professionals are to be found way down in the organisation's hierarchy.

Proactive use of in–house expertise is also important in pushing towards best practice standards. Risk management expertise, including health, safety and environmental specialists, should not just be consulted when there is a problem, but when plans and developments are being considered so that problems can be avoided.

Establishing effective systems   6.57

Prior to the publication of HSE's *Successful Health and Safety Management* in 1991, (updated in 1997),[2] a specialist part of the HSE had spent over 15 years carrying out detailed reviews of health and safety management systems in an extensive number of employing organisations. Many of these organisations were at the leading edge in terms of effective systems to manage health, safety and environmental risks. The HSE guidance therefore reflected in some detail what organisations in practice did to achieve enviable health and safety performance. This background is important to appreciate because it adds to the weight of this particular HSE publication. The guidance describes a five-step management system (see **FIGURE 6.1**).

Figure 6.1: The five-step cycle

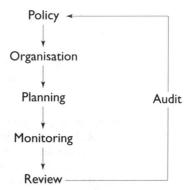

The steps in the system constitute an iterative process which is repeated over time in order to secure progressively better performance. The steps are similar to general approaches developed more recently in relation to controls assurance and corporate governance. Health and safety professionals have been known to debate where in the loop an organisation needs to start. It is, however, fair to say that in the absence of policy, an organisational structure and plans, it is not possible to carry out the successive parts of the loop in a meaningful way. It therefore makes sense to start with policy and work through the other steps in a logical fashion.

A typical situation   6.58

Anyone who has stepped into a risk management role within a healthcare organisation will, however, know from experience that typically:

- Some policies exist, but they are not up to date, the chief executive has forgotten to sign them, and many parts of the organisation have never seen them. Others have seen them but do not follow them.

- Some semblance of an organisational structure is in place, but there is often lack of clarity about the roles of groups and individuals, so that much effort is duplicated and other issues are not addressed at all.

- Health and safety planning consists of reacting to events that happen, and earmarking a percentage of the budget for health and safety but failing to prioritise how the money is spent.

- Monitoring performance is normally reactive and only consists of reviewing recorded incidents. Active monitoring of achievement of planned objectives is rare.

- Performance review is rarely done in-house and most usually involves consultants, CNST assessors, NAO staff, financial auditors or HSE inspectors.

With some effort, this scenario can be turned around so that the healthcare organisation drives its health and safety programme rather than the other way round!

The five-step process
Policies   6.59

These do not need to be lengthy documents which cover every conceivable angle. Many multinational organisations employing thousands of people throughout the world succeed in producing health, safety and environmental policies which cover no more than one side of A4.

Aim for a short general policy document which sets out the organisation's overall aspirations and key responsibilities of individuals.

The general policy can be supplemented by other policies dealing with specific areas of risk such as infection control, laboratory work, and directorate policies. Some points to remember are:

- The policy should be signed by the organisation head, dated and regularly reviewed.

151

- It should recognise that health, safety and the environment is central to high quality service delivery, reducing costs and looking after staff.

- Be wary of including large slices of legal requirements in a policy document as this is meaningless in conveying aspirations.

- Include positive statements about why health and safety is important.

- Make sure that the policy can be read and easily understood by all groups of staff.

Forward-looking health and safety policies reflect the need to develop people and become an integral part of ensuring organisational success and effective staff development. Policies increasingly recognise the continuum between work life and non-work life and that an individual's performance, and in consequence that of the employing organisation, is affected by work and non-work experiences.

Organisation   6.60

The overall aim should be to implement the health and safety policy and to facilitate the move to better performance.

Good organisation involves assigning responsibilities to those members of staff with key health and safety responsibilities and also groups, such as the health and safety committee, risk management group and manual handling coordinators.

Organisational arrangements need to ensure that:

- The organisation drives its health and safety programme – not the other way round.

- Cooperation is encouraged and not hampered.

- Staff are competent and undertake roles assigned to them.

- There is effective communication from the top down, the bottom up and throughout all layers of the organisation.

Planning   6.61

This should be viewed as the means by which priorities and objectives are established in relation to health, safety and environmental risks. Risk assessment and incident analysis are a key part of planning, in order that priorities are properly set. Planning is about proactivity and deciding what to do next on the basis of available evidence.

Effective planning requires resources to be assigned, teamworking and a desire to see progress happen. It requires determination and commitment. Objectives for improvement need to be SMART: specific, measurable, achievable, realistic and time-bound. A good test of effective planning is to ask whether there is an overall plan for health, safety and environmental issues and whether the right priorities are indicated in the plan.

Monitoring   6.62

Monitoring progress and measuring performance are key steps in ensuring increasing improvement in performance over time. Health and safety professionals often categorise monitoring systems as either active or reactive. Incident recording is in essence reactive monitoring; active monitoring is more concerned with the achievement of plans. Examples of active monitoring of progress include:

- attendance by staff at a risk assessment training course;

- appointment of manual handling coordinators; and

- refurbishment of the gas-scavenging system in theatres.

In other words, active monitoring is about checking achievement of specific objectives in the health and safety plan.

Review and audit   6.63

The previous four steps form the main plank of a health and safety management system, but it is important to check that the system is having the desired effect in terms of health and safety performance. This brings us to the review step. This step encompasses the use of audits, of which there are many in the health and safety arena.

Many organisations outside of the healthcare sector place regular reliance on health and safety audits to verify their performance. These audits are either carried out in-house or by external consultants. Some audits are paper-based, others software-based. Some have been developed specifically for the healthcare sector. In purchasing a proprietary audit package, of which there are several, it is important to establish that the audit is relevant and is capable of being repeatedly used over a period of time. This is a specialist area and one where the views of health and safety colleagues should be sought.

Stress   6.64

Stress is expensive, for both organisations and individuals, as it can lead to sickness absence, reduced performance at work, long term ill-health, redeployment and premature retirement. HSE defines work-related stress as 'the adverse reaction people have to excessive pressures or other types of demand placed upon them'.[10] This definition appears not to recognize that under-utilisation at work 'rust out' in American parlance can also be a source of stress although this is unlikely to be a widespread problem in the healthcare sector.

Stress is a normal feature of life. It is necessary to motivate individuals to 'go the extra mile' or rise to the occasion that a new challenge brings. Up to a point, stress is therefore beneficial and an aspect of job satisfaction. The difficulty for managers is to judge the point at which it is no longer beneficial varies between individuals because people respond differently to stress. Some seem to thrive on tough work goals and tight deadlines, while others cope less well. The affect of work-related stress is intertwined with stress in an individual's personal life. Financial problems, family bereavement, divorce and other major adult life experiences can all be a source of stress which can affect the ability to cope with pressure in the working environment. All of this makes managing stress in the workplace one of the most difficult tasks for managers.

There is no specific health and safety legislation in connection with stress at work. However, the *HSWA 1974* requires employers to ensure the health of their employees at work. The *Management Regulations 1999 (SI 1999/3242)* include duties to assess risks to health, implement measures to prevent exposure to risk and provide training. These general legal requirements apply to stress in the same way that they apply to other aspects of work that can affect health such as exposure to chemicals.

Stress in the healthcare sector   6.65

Within the healthcare sector, stress can arise from long hours of work, unsociable shift patterns and interrupted rest and meal breaks. Further contributing factors include:

- the threat of violence and aggression;

- the emotional toll of dealing with sick and dying patients;

- being personally blamed for incidents;

- unexpected patient outcomes; and

- being the subject of patient complaint.

The constant reorganisation and reconfiguration of health service bodies and the establishment of more organisations which set targets for and monitor the performance of healthcare providers compounds the stress which arises from day to day activities.

Towards the end of 2003, HSE served an Improvement Notice on a NHS trust in the West Country. HSE considered that the mental health trust had inadequate procedures to assess the risk of stress among staff. The notice required that risk assessments were undertaken to assess the exposure of staff to stress at work. Enforcement action by HSE in relation to stress is unusual, but this is likely to increase as this is a priority topic for HSE in the healthcare sector. It is intended that HSC's Health Services Advisory Committee (HSAC) publishes guidance on work-related stress, based upon a research project undertaken by HSE in conjunction with the trade

union UNISON and the (Royal College of Nursing) RCN. The guidance is anticipated in 2004.[11]

Dealing with stress 6.66

HSE has produced a useful managers' guide to tackling stress.[12] This is a pack of
documents which includes:

- Two guidance books for managers on how to comply with legal requirements.

- A guidance leaflet for employees.

- An action planner.

- Prompt cards to help pin-point possible solutions to stress problems.

- A series of case studies giving practical examples of measure undertaken to
  deal with work-related stress.

Healthcare managers and directors will find the document pack useful as several
of the case studies are relevant to the healthcare sector. Case studies include a hospital, a NHS trust, a care home, social services, violence, role ambiguity and conflict in the public sector.

The risk assessment process described earlier (**SEE 6.11 TO 6.18**) can be applied to
work-related stress; in essence this is what is required by health and safety legislation. In practice this requires consideration of a number of organisational features,
including:

- Culture.

- Management style.

- Work patterns and demands.

- Working relationships.

- Role clarity.

- How well staff are equipped to undertake their roles.

- Day to day support between colleagues and from managers.

- Professional support such as counselling.

Many organisations have now undertaken stress surveys amongst their staff, sometimes developed in conjunction with external stress experts, to identify the extent
and location of stress. Well constructed surveys produce valuable information,
which when combined with sickness and absence data, staff turnover and performance data can highlight where problems lie. The information can be analysed to
identify what action is merited to tackle stress. Often the evidence confirms that a
particular individual is a source of significant stress for colleagues. If this is the

case, it is important for organisations to address the problem irrespective of whether it is a board member, senior manager or a junior member of staff that is implicated.

Violence and aggression   6.67

The threat of violence and aggression in the healthcare sector is a well recognised and increasing problem. Many surveys and reviews have drawn attention to the scale of the problem, the circumstances in which it may arise and the steps that can be taken to reduce the chance of staff being adversely affected.[13] In the main violence and aggression towards healthcare staff is perpetrated by patients, members of patients' families and their friends. Aggressive and bullying behaviour between members of staff does also take place.

Research has shown that:

- Physical assaults to NHS staff are the third largest cause of accidents resulting in more than three days of absence.

- Nurses experience the highest risk of assault after security personnel.

- In 2001–2002 there were 84,000 reported incidents of violence and aggression against healthcare staff.

Tackling violence   6.68

HSE has taken forward a number of initiatives to tackle violence and aggression in the healthcare sector. In 1997, they produced specific guidance on assessing the risks to healthcare staff and management interventions to reduce risk.[14] Since 1996 HSE has given priority to violence and aggression within their inspections of healthcare premises. Local activity has involved the development of training material for trusts and their partner organisations.[15] At the end of the last decade, the NHS introduced the zero tolerance campaign in order to increase public understanding that violence against NHS staff would not be tolerated. More recent developments include the decisions by some trusts to withhold treatment and care from aggressive and violent patients. In January 2003, the Counter Fraud and Security Management Service was created as a new Special Health Authority. Part of its remit includes violence in the healthcare sector and an early initiative has been the introduction of a conflict resolution training programme for NHS staff.

For healthcare organisations to effectively tackle this problem, a number of measures need to be in place:

- Incident recording systems need to be able to capture episodes of violence and aggression.

- Staff must be encouraged and feel free to report.

- The involvement of the police should be considered in the investigation of incidents and in the development of prevention strategies.

- Staff must be trained to recognize the signs of aggressive behaviour, in the use of de-escalation skills and in the techniques of control and restraint.

- Risk assessments should be completed.

- Physical measures such as CCTVs, personal alarms and the improved design and layout of working areas should be in place as dictated by risk assessment.

The progress that trusts are making to implement these improvements has been reviewed by the NAO.[16] In this review report produced in 2003 the NAO touched on the difficulty of determining the costs to the NHS of violence and aggression. A crude estimate of £69 million per annum has been suggested as the direct cost to the NHS. This tentative figure is likely to be a significant under-estimation because of the extent of under-reporting of this area of risk. The costs alone ought to be sufficient to encourage managers to introduce easy to use reporting systems and the precautions necessary to prevent this type of harm to staff.

Healthcare staff must resist the temptation to see violence and aggression as a normal part of their working day. In reality, however, staff in A&E may find it easier to be less tolerant of such behaviour than those caring for elderly, confused or disabled patients. Nonetheless it is entirely reasonable for healthcare employers to set out acceptable standards of conduct by patients and to make clear the outcome should the standard not be met. No one should reach home at the end of a day's work physically or psychologically damaged, especially those employed in the caring professions.

Occupational health 6.69

Many of the risks that healthcare workers face in their day to day activities are associated with the potential for their health to be adversely affected. It is therefore important that there are adequate arrangements for occupational health (OH) service provision not just to support HR colleagues but to reduce exposure to health risks at work and to provide specialist support should a work-related problem arise.

Irrespective of whether the OH service is provided under contract by an external organisation or by an in-house team, it should encompass the range of support that the healthcare organisation needs. Many organisations both within and outside the healthcare sector, determine their OH needs with little consideration of the nature and extent of the health risks faced by staff. This leads to health issues being inadequately addressed and often a loss of confidence in the OH service by staff and managers. The best way forward prior to appointing OH providers or re-scoping the existing service, is for a needs analysis to be undertaken; this ought to include consideration of risk assessments, reported incidents and work practices which have lead or have the potential to lead to work-related ill health. Only then can the precise expertise that the OH service needs to be able to provide be determined. An organisational needs analysis will enable decisions to be made about:

- The amount of OH physician cover whether full time or weekly sessions.

- The number of OH nurses and the nature of their expertise.

- The need for and amount of physiotherapy support.

- Access to ergonomic expertise.

- The provision of stress counselling.

- Occupational hygiene requirements for monitoring work place exposure.

- Whether the service should be kept in-house or out-sourced or a combination of the two.

OH service provision in healthcare should not be restricted to pre-employment assessments, vaccination of staff, dealing with self and management referrals and contributing to decisions about redeployment and early retirement of staff. For the health of staff to be protected it is necessary for OH service providers to be pro-active, so that they contribute to the development of safe working practices and risk assessments, give advice about how harm can be prevented, develop policies on key health issues and audit actual working practices. Sadly, it is often the case that the OH service provider does not have the resources to provide a more pro-active service and may indeed be restricted from doing so by the contract for OH service provision. It should therefore be that the manager of the service recognizes the need for pro-activity, initiates a needs analysis and then pulls together a team which is appropriately sized and has the required areas of expertise. The composition of the team should be kept under review as particular problems are dealt with and other priorities are identified. OH service provision lends itself to short term injections of expertise to enable specific problems to be tackled.

One of the issues faced by in-house OH service providers in trusts is the expectation for income generation. Whilst this may be beneficial in broadening the experience of the members of the OH team it can create further pressure on an already stretched team. In such situations the standard of support to the host organisation usually suffers. In many instances the revenue generated from providing support to other organisations is not retained within the OH budget. The provision of OH support to other organisations by healthcare OH service providers does increase the number of people who have access to OH services but the breadth and quality of the cover may suffer in consequence.

For health and safety risks to be adequately managed in any large organisation, there needs to be an effective working relationship between the OH and safety specialists. In reality this is often not the case. Different reporting lines, crowded work agendas, lack of awareness of respective areas of expertise and sometimes role conflict and hostility can all conspire for a less than harmonious and effective working relationship. It is possible that the health of employees may suffer as a result together with the quality of decision making in relation to work-related ill health matters. This can be avoided if OH and safety specialists:

• understand their respective areas of expertise;

• work together to solve problems;

• recognize that they each have an important part to play in improving the health of employees;

• resolve a means to communicate on health and safety performance data such as recorded incidents, RIDDOR notifications and cases of work-related ill health;

• are co-located within the same building or at least nearby; and

• conduct regular liaison meetings to review progress on agreed action and discuss progress on work-related matters.

Improving OH in the healthcare sector   6.70

In 1994, HSAC produced a number of objectives for the healthcare sector.[7] One of those objectives related to the availability of OH (and safety) services for all healthcare staff and that the service would have the full confidence of staff. HSAC's overall aim was that this and other improvements would be in place across the healthcare sector within ten years. The ten year deadline is now with us and in many healthcare organisations has not been achieved. The challenges for OH service providers have increased since 1994 as in 2000 the Health and Safety Commission launched a further initiative – *Securing Health Together*.[9] This was an OH strategy for Great Britian which contained a number or targets (SEE **6.55**).

In relation to these targets it is worth considering how many healthcare organisations together with their OH service can actually determine the base levels for these targets let alone identify progress in relation to their achievement. HSC recognized that these targets would not be met over night and that a series of actions and changes would need to be implemented for reductions to become apparent. They may not have appreciated just how much progress needed to be made in the healthcare sector in relation to the management of work-related health risks and the challenge of applying the targets to patients.

In 2003, the NAO conducted a review of the management of health and safety risks to staff in NHS trusts. The subsequent NAO report[16] looked at progress in reducing the extent and costs of accidents to staff and the management of specific health and safety risks. In relation to OH service provision, the NAO found that few trusts routinely analysed ill health data to determine priorities and that OH staff tended to react to problems that had arisen. The review also identified that OH staff were often dissatisfied with the geographical location of their department, the quality of and space afforded by their accommodation and the lack of OH resources. Despite the problems identified by the NAO, it is to be hoped that healthcare organisations and OH specialists will however rise to the challenge and help make health and safety performance across the healthcare sector a model for others to emulate as envisaged by HSAC in 1994.[7]

Interface with clinical risk   6.71

When the healthcare sector first started to give priority to risk management, clinical and non-clinical risk tended to be separated. There were a number of reasons for this. Different individuals, particularly within hospitals, were responsible for these areas. The absence of a coordinated risk management strategy also contributed to the separation. Clinical risk tended to be regarded as the preserve of clinicians, and non-clinical risk the responsibility of others.

Within hospitals the use of different incident recording systems to record clinical and non-clinical incidents, and the fact that the number and nature of these incidents were rarely combined for scrutiny, also played its part. The healthcare sector lost valuable ground in dealing with risk management by allowing clinical and non-clinical risk to be separated. Within the health and safety profession in general there is considerable expertise in incident recording, analysis, trend spotting, root cause analysis and implementing change when things have gone wrong. This expertise can be deployed in looking at incidents in general, including clinical incidents. Even now in many parts of the healthcare sector the separation between clinical and non-clinical risk still exists. The DoH's report *An Organisation with a Memory* (SEE **KEY REFERENCES, APPENDIX 1**) and the diversity of expertise tapped into during the preparation of the report clearly illustrate the benefits of involving risk experts from outside the clinical arena.

Recent HSE prosecutions   6.72

Over the last couple of years, there have been a number of prosecutions taken by HSE inspectors as a consequence of hospital incidents. On first examination these incidents, some of which have been described earlier in this chapter (SEE **6.28** AND **6.30**), would appear to be clinical incidents in which patients have either been harmed or even killed. The HSE has, however, succeeded in demonstrating to the criminal courts that health and safety legislation nonetheless applies, and healthcare providers have been accordingly convicted of breaches of this legislation. This has further called into question the wisdom of separating clinical and non-clinical risk.

The HSC has reviewed the arrangements for enforcing *section 3* of the *HSWA 1974* in relation to patient safety and more broadly. This lead, in January 2004, to the signing of a Memorandum of Understanding between HSE and the GMC in relation to respective roles and responsibilities for patient safety.[17]

One case that illustrates the lack of wisdom in separating clinical and non-clinical risk is an HSE prosecution which followed the death of a patient undergoing a cardiac angiogram described above (SEE **6.28**). The important point about this case is that many lessons can be learnt not just in relation to clinical practice, but in relation to managing risk more broadly. The successful HSE prosecution serves to underline the importance of looking at incidents on a more holistic basis and the difficulties which may arise if approaches to clinical and non-clinical risk are compartmentalised.

References

1   HSE (1998) *Five Steps to Risk Assessment*, Health & Safety Executive, London.
2   HSE (1997) *Successful Health & Safety Management*, Health & Safety Executive, London.
3   Mayatt VL (1997) *HSE prosecutes NHS trust*, Sedgwick Insight Volume 10 Issue 6
4   The Courier January 29 2004. www.thecourier.co.uk
5   Forlin G (2001) *Corporate killing: where are we now?* Proceedings of the 2001 IOSH Conference.
6   Mayatt VL (1996) 'The management of occupational health and safety', *Health Care Risk Report*, vol 2, no 10.
7   HSC Health Service Advisory Committee (1994) *Management of health and safety in the health services – information for managers and directors*. HMSO.
8   HSE (2000) *Revitalising Health and Safety*, Health & Safety Executive, London.
9   HSE (2000) *Securing health together*, Health & Safety Executive, London.
10 HSE (2003) *Tackling work-related stress. A managers' guide to improving and maintaining employee health and well-being.*
11 HSC (2003) *Delivering health and safety in Great Britain*. HSC annual report for 2002–2003.
12 HSE (2003) *Real solutions, real people. A managers' guide to tackling work-related stress.*
13 Mayatt V L (2003) 'Violence and aggression: not part of the working day', *Health Care Risk Report*, vol 9, issue 7.
14 HSC Health Service Advisory Committee (1997) *Violence and aggression to staff in the health services*, HMSO.
15 Mayatt VL (2003) 'Nurses assaulted by violent client', *Health Care Risk Report*, vol 9, issue 9.
16 NAO (2003) *A safer place to work, protecting NHS hospital and ambulance staff from violence and aggression.*
17 http://www.hse.gov.uk/aboutus/framework/mou/gmc-mou.pdf

Further information

HSE Direct: www.hsedirect.com

Health at Work in the NHS (*www.hawnhs.hda-online.org.uk*)

BMA (1994) *Environmental and Occupational Risks of Healthcare*, BMA publishing, London.

HSE (1998) *Guide to Risk Assessment Requirements*, Health & Safety Executive, London.

HSE (1996) *The Costs of Accidents at Work*, Health & Safety Executive, London.

HSE (2003) *Occupational Exposure Limits*, Health & Safety Executive, London.

Health Services Advisory Committee (1997), *The Management of Occupational Health Services for Healthcare Staff*, HSAC, Luton.

Health Services Advisory Committee (1998), *Manual handing in the health services*

Harrington JM, Gill FS, Aw TC and Gardiner K (1998), *Occupational health*, Blackwell Science

Chapter 7
Managing the Physical Environment

This chapter covers:

- The healthcare physical environment.

- Estates and facilities management (EfM).

- Estates and facilities services in healthcare Private Finance Initiatives (PFI).

- Contracting for facilities management service delivery.

- Facilities operational risk: pressure systems, maintenance, fire, and electricity.

- Security of staff and assets.

- Training and development.

Introduction   7.1

The physical or built environment is increasingly recognised as a vital component of the provision of effective healthcare. There are more than 700 safety-related statutes in the UK, and approximately 100 of these are of day-to-day concern to those providing services and running facilities management and estates functions in healthcare establishments.

In addition there are over 100 authoritative codes of practice – and with guidance constantly growing or being updated, it is vital that facilities staff remain well briefed on statutory compliance and risk management. There are a large number of statutory issues affecting facilities management (FM), along with a number of controls assurance standards (see **KEY REFERENCES, APPENDIX 1**). This chapter will outline some of the major areas for property-related statutory compliance, and key aspects of facilities risk that relate to FM services and the physical environment.

The provision of healthcare is a holistic process which combines the three elements of people (staff), process (work patterns, routines and systems) and workplace. Clearly the physical environment (building or hospital) needs to support the activity or process that takes place within it and be fit for purpose, whilst providing an environment that is warm, comfortable, clean, attractive and safe for staff, patients and visitors. A therapeutic and supportive physical environment can have a positive effect on recuperation and also the morale of patients, staff and visitors.

A varied environment 7.2

The physical environment in which healthcare is delivered can vary greatly in terms of size, age, design, decorative order and condition. Modern hospitals and healthcare establishments are designed and built in line with Health Building Notes which provide guidance on the design and layout of specialist areas and infrastructure to support effective service delivery, such as intensive care units and theatres. Healthcare space standards and departmental cost allowance guidance (DCAG) now reflect consumerism requirements and reflect the additional space required to provide highly serviced healthcare environments which match up to patient expectation in ward and clinical areas. Clinical links and departmental interdependencies are now considered at the design stage in new healthcare developments, in order to ensure that typical patient journeys are taken into account and that the building supports the delivery of healthcare and the patient journey requirements

The patient journey 7.3

The patient journey details the route map that the patient follows during a particular episode of treatment, and outlines all of the areas, services and clinical specialties that they may encounter until the episode is completed. This approach takes into account typical patient flow patterns, maps contact with specialist departments and establishes how often, where and when the patient encounters these services.

By taking into account these regular and routine interactions, the hospital can be designed or redesigned in such a way as to support typical patient journeys. This in turn avoids unnecessary patient movement, and logistical problems where staff and vital equipment have to be moved around the hospital or find themselves inappropriately located. Older healthcare premises may have been developed without full consideration to the patient journey or interdependency.

The challenge of older buildings 7.4

Due to the changing nature of healthcare delivery methods, a large number of hospitals and healthcare premises have outlived their original design concepts, and are not suitable to support the provision of modern healthcare services which are high-tech and highly serviced. This presents risk relating to service provision.

The NHS has the largest property portfolio in Europe comprising some 1,200 hospital sites worth around £23 billion. Sixty-five per cent of the estate is over 35 years old, with a large number of Victorian and listed properties. A large amount of the NHS estate was not designed to support today's methods of healthcare delivery. New technology and healthcare tecniques cannot be supported in these outdated properties and in many instances, the physical layout of the site and buildings do not support effective and supportive patient journeys. Significant investment has been made on making these bulidings compliant with fire safety and the *Disability Discrimination Act 1995* (DDA). The NHS Plan (see **KEY REF-ERENCES, APPENDIX 1**) sets a target that 40% of the total NHS building stock will be less than 15 years old by 2010, and 25% of the NHS maintenance backlog will be cleared by 2004. Much of this backlog maintenance reduction will be achieved by the provision of 100 new hospitals by 2010 (mostly provided under PFI arangements). In turn this will mean a large part of the existing estate and associated backlog maintenance will be reduced or demolished (as part of redevelopment) or sold on as part of the sale of the surplus NHS property portfolio.

A large amount of the current NHS estate has significant backlog maintenance and robust risk management is required in order to manage risk relating to issues such as fire safety, Legionella, asbestos, *DDA 1995* and electricity. There are also a number of other risk factors that need to be addressed – business risk, service continuity, outsourcing, procurement of services and contract management all fall into this important category.

NHS Estates and the HSE are seriously concerned about the risks posed by the large quantity (thousands of tonnes) of asbestos materials that may be present in healthcare buildings. It is essential that asbestos be effectively managed, particularly with the drive to modernise and upgrade or even dispose of premises as the risk of disturbing or exposing asbestos may be heightened as a result. A new duty has been introduced into the *Control of Asbestos at Work Regulations 2002 (SI 2002/2675)*, which requires those organisations with a responsibility for maintenance activities, to manage the risk from asbestos in their buildings.

Old or new, the property, people and process combination needs to be carefully and effectively managed with respect to risk, including health and safcty. Risk needs to be assessed and managed in the buildings in use, the processes or work methods followed, and in the management of staff, patients and visitors within the healthcare environment.

Estates and facilities management   7.5

The term 'facilities management' is still a relatively new concept to healthcare. There is no standard model of service provision, so the basket of services managed under the FM umbrella and the links to the trust board vary widely. Unlike Finance and Medical Directors there is no compulsion to have a Director of Estates or Facilities on the executive team or trust board and this can limit the ability to address estates issues in a strategic manner. The growth of FM in UK healthcare over the past decade has been rapid and far-reaching. The facilities profession has developed from its early formative stage in the late 1980s, through a rapid growth phase during the 1990s. It is reaching a level of maturity and credibility which will guide it through the first decade of the new millennium.

Facilities service contractors   7.6

Similarly, the majority of facilities service contractors have gone through a meta-morphic change over the last few years. Many companies have been acquired by or merged with large construction firms, while large-scale professional cleaning contractors have acquired catering contract companies with the aim of extending the basket of services that they can offer. The overall result has been the emergence of a 'super league' of facilities providers who can cover the broad remit of healthcare facilities and estates management.

These service providers are able to service a wide market apart from healthcare, including sectors such as education, defence and local government. Some of these FM providers are now poised to take on global FM. They are also positioning themselves as consortium partners for the Private Finance Initiative (PFI) and Public/Private Partnerships (PPP) – deals that will secure contracts for periods of 25–35 years. As the healthcare sector matures, many PFI FM providers are now investing equity into PFI/PPP deals.

The professionals involved   7.7

The evolution of FM has involved professionals from a varied collection of professional disciplines in the management of facilities services. Property and the built environment play a key role and this has required the professional skills of architects and quantity surveyors. The way that people interact with the built environment has required the input of human resources professionals and the technical expertise of building services and maintenance staff.

The processes that take place within buildings such as catering, cleaning, security, or the mailroom have required practical operational management from a range of specialist professional backgrounds – not to forget the overriding management of risk across all of the disciplines. This varied assortment of professional and management skills, coupled with pressure to downsize the organisation and to flatten management hierarchy, has spawned a new breed – the facilities manager.

The new breed of facilities manager   7.8

The new breed of facilities manager is likely to be responsible for a range of services outside their original professional discipline. It is commonplace for those who used to be quantity surveyors, architects, maintenance engineers, office managers, catering managers and human resource managers to now be responsible for the delivery of the full range of facilities services in their organisation. Facilities managers have by necessity become generalists not specialists. This, however, should not in itself present a risk management or service management issue. Healthcare FM is after all predominately a management function – which achieves its results by harnessing the effective output from people, property and process.

Defining FM   7.9

Many definitions of FM exist but they are all variations on a theme. The following definition of FM, from NHS Estates, will be used and expanded upon in this chapter:

> 'The practice of coordinating the physical workplace with the people and work of an organisation; [FM] integrates the principles of business administration, architecture, and the behavioural and engineering sciences.'

A core function   7.10

The traditional view of FM has been that of a non-core or pure support function which is often seen to be at arm's length to the main thrust of activities of the organisation. From a risk management perspective, it is vital that each organisation understands the importance of facilities services and fully considers the services it deems to be core and non-core to its operation.

Certainly, in the early days of FM, much emphasis was placed upon facilities taking control of and managing all of the non-critical or non-core functions – which would then enable the organisation to focus on the main business agenda and the core issues that it might be facing. Clearly there are benefits associated with combining the management of support functions under one umbrella. Additional benefit is achieved by breaking down traditional demarcation boundaries and combining service functions in an innovative manner – cutting out duplication and wasteful practice.

The extent of FM   7.11

Many organisations are now beginning to realise the true potential of FM services and recognise that they are more than just pure support functions limited to operational service delivery. The evolving nature of FM and the maturity of its approach has begun to ensure that a strategic FM dimension is now a requirement for all successful and forward-thinking organisations.

If all the functions of a healthcare organisation were to be analysed and the processes involved portrayed as a supply chain, then a number of key links in the chain would be provided and managed by the facilities function. In its best operational mode, FM could be described as the glue that holds the organisation together. The FM span covers tasks achieved by basic manual handling at one end of the spectrum, through to hi-tech, highly-serviced electronic medical devices at the other.

Facilities strategy   7.12

As FM has evolved and developed within organisations, there has been a steady realisation of the benefits (tangible and intangible) that can be obtained from effective management of FM services. If facilities professionals are to be truly regarded as players within the organisation, then it is essential for the facilities manager to develop a facilities strategy. This should map over a stated period of time how FM services will be reviewed, re-engineered or moulded to best support the needs of the organisation.

The strategy should ideally comprise three strategic elements that build upon the current level of provision and should map short, medium and long-term goals and targets and give direction for facilities over the stated period. If the strategy is to be of any real value then it must reflect the aims and ambitions of the organisation that it is designed to support. The facilities strategy must clearly complement the overriding business strategy, and this can only happen if the senior facilities professional is in tune with the vision of the organisation.

A thorough approach to risk management underpins service delivery and should be outlined in a way that is clearly understood in the facilities strategy. As the organisation evolves over time the strategic direction may need to be modified to take account of external influencing factors, which will require emergent strategy to be developed – this approach may also mean that elements of strategy remain unrealised (SEE FIGURE 7.1).

Figure 7.1: Strategy development

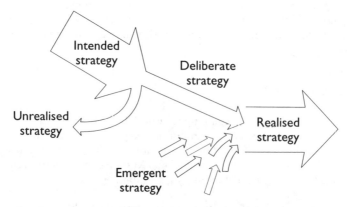

The developed strategy must, however, take account of the core business of the organisation and its own corporate strategy, direction, mission and values. If FM is to develop in harmony with the organisation that it supports, then it must develop a degree of strategic alignment and focus upon shared values. Also, more importantly, the facilities manager must become a part of the decision-making body (that is, a board-level player) if facilities are truly to become proactive and to ensure that the full risk impact of facilities-related issues are considered.

Facilities risk 7.13

Facilities risk can be focused into two specific areas:

- **Strategic risk** – risks associated with procuring service contracts, including out-sourcing and in-sourcing decisions.

- **Operational risks** – risks associated with day-to-day operational provision of a range of facilities services, many of which are covered by statutory legislation and guidance.

Contracting for facilities management

European procurement process 7.14

Public procurement law states that any public service contract with a sum total in excess of the relevant threshold must comply with European Union General Agreement on Tariffs and Trade (GATT) legislation when going out to the market to test services. Compliance with the EU Directive on public procurement is mandatory. Its Directive is to promote and maintain competition in public procurement within the EU, to control restrictive practices, and to try to create a level playing field for potential contractors competing for work.

There are three procedure options:

- restricted;

- open; and

- negotiated.

Restricted procedure 7.15

Restricted procedure is most frequently used within the NHS, and enables the selection of tenders to be controlled. The contracting authority invites interested parties to show Expressions of Interest and from the received expressions a selected group is invited to tender.

Information note number 14/03 dated 9/12/03 detailed the revision of EC and Government Procurement Agreement (GPA) procurement thresholds, see Table 7.1.

Table 7.1: Thresholds – public sector from 1 January 2004

	Supplies	Services	Works
Entities listed in Schedule[1] (SI 1995/201)	£99,695 (SDR130,000) (€154,014)	£99,695[2] (SDR130,000) (€154,014)	£99,695[3] (SDR130,000) (€154,014)
Other public sector contracting authorities	£153,376 (SDR200,000) (€236,945)	£153,376[2] (SDR200,000) (€236,945)	£3,834,411[3] (SDR5,000,000) (€5,923,624)
Indicative Notices	£485,481 (€750,000)	£485,481 (€750,000)	£3,834,411 (€5,923,624)
Small Lots	Not applicable	£51,785 (€80,000)	£647,308 (€1,000,000)

1   *Schedule 1* of the *Public Supply Contracts Regulations 1995 (SI 1995/201)* lists central Government bodies. These thresholds will also apply to any successor bodies.
2   With the exception of the following services, which have a threshold of £129,462 (€200,000):
  ● Part B (residual) services
  ● Research and Development Services (Category 8)
  ● The following Telecommunications services in Category 5
    ○ CPC 7524 – Television and Radio Broadcast services
    ○ CPC 7525 – Interconnection services
    ○ CPC 7526 – Integrated telecommunications services
  ● Subsidised services contracts under *regulation 25* of the *Public Services Contracts Regulations 1993 (SI 1993/3228)*.
3   For subsidised works contracts under *regulation 23* of the *Public Works Contracts Regulations 1991 (SI 1991/2680)* and Works Concessions the threshold is £3,236,542 (€5,000,000).

All contracts exceeding a stated threshold value (excluding VAT) must be advertised in the *Official Journal of the European Community* (OJEC) for a period of 37 days prior to the Invitation to Tender. Tenders must be issued for a period of not less than 40 days to those responding within 48 days of a contract award, and notification must be placed in the OJEC. Selection of tenders from those responding to the advertisement must not discriminate on grounds of nationality. Criteria for exclusion are specific and organisations must be able to demonstrate fairness in the selection process.

Open procedure   7.16

Open procedure is also available but is less frequently used, as it allows all of those expressing an interest to receive tenders and has a longer period (52 days) for receipt of Expressions of Interest.

Negotiated procedure   7.17

Negotiated procedure involves direct discussion and negotiation between supplier and procurer in order to arrive at a final offer. This procedure requires careful consideration as it attracts ministerial attention, and there needs to be clear reasons why the negotiated route has been chosen over the open and restricted options. It is therefore only available in limited circumstances.

Exemptions to the procedures   7.18

Bearing in mind the purpose of the legislation, exemptions are limited and strictly defined. In the case of genuine urgency (failure to plan ahead is specifically excluded) an accelerated procedure may be allowed – an example might be the sudden and unforeseeable failure of a critical piece of equipment, but not an unexpected release of funds.

Where appropriate, the period for receipt of Expressions of Interest may be reduced to 15 days and the tender period to 10 days.

Non-compliance   7.19

Where suppliers feel that they have been unfairly disadvantaged they are encouraged to seek redress through the *Compliance Directive* (a section of the *EU Directive on public procurement*). Therefore in any circumstances where a supplier is excluded from competition, the reasons must be set down and must be applied equally to all suppliers.

The Government requires an annual return from all public bodies showing the value of business placed within and outside the Directives. Failure to comply with the legislation is likely to be noticed.

The decision to outsource   7.20

The decision to outsource elements of an organisation's facilities activity or support service delivery is a major strategic decision. The ultimate decision must be based on confidence that the service provider can deliver a consistent, affordable, high-quality service in accordance with the specification, whilst demonstrating synergy with the future strategic direction of the host organisation. The decision will be based upon a key set of circumstances usually focused around cost, quality, service delivery and risk – unique in each instance and for each organisation, often with each factor weighted to reflect impact and importance.

Clearing dead wood   7.21

Charles Handy wrote:[1]

> 'Organisations are responding to the challenge of efficiency by exporting unproductive work and people as fast as they can.'

171

It is true to say that some of the early outsourcing decisions were made for all of the wrong reasons. Rather than tackling or managing issues relating to lack of flexibility, generic working methods or rigid demarcation boundaries, many organisations outsourced what they considered to be inflexible and uncooperative departments and service functions.

In so doing, unruly management and supervision were transferred to the outsourced provider for them to manage and control. For many organisations, outsourcing was initially seen as an opportunity to clear the dead wood and reduce headcount, fuelled by a trend towards downsizing. The decision to outsource may also have been influenced by a focus on the complexity of day-to-day service issues without perhaps considering some of the longer-term issues.

Careful consideration   7.22

What do organisations gain from outsourcing? The decision to outsource or in-source must be thoroughly considered and evaluated before a decision is made. Outsourcing or in-sourcing can have a demoralising impact on staff groups and result in a reduction of output and productivity in the short term.

If the original decision to outsource was wrong then this may lead an organisation to consider bringing the service back in-house. Often by the time this point has been reached, a considerable pool of labour, expertise, loyalty and knowledge has been lost as a result of the initial transition and this will make returning to in-sourcing more difficult. This does not make it impossible, but there will undoubtedly be a time lag whilst the service re-establishes itself and expertise is developed. A hump of costs associated with setting up human resources, payroll, management and supervisory structures will be incurred as systems are put back into place.

Core versus non-core   7.23

The core versus non-core discussion should be considered in the outsourcing debate, in order to determine the services that the organisation retains or manages in-house. Careful consideration needs to be given to identifying those services that are best managed directly by the organisation.

A strategic view must be established on the importance of each service element when it comes to risk and business continuity. It is important to identify knowledge in each service area, to establish the value of that knowledge and to gauge how difficult it would be to replicate each function. It is therefore vital that the functional linkages and service boundaries that exist between departments and directorates are identified and mapped, before any contract bundle or service package is assembled prior to outsourcing.

Talk over lunch   7.24

In most organisations there are often casual arrangements in place between departments to resolve minor issues, such as discussion over lunch of minor problems. This interaction happens on an informal but regular basis and is never in the specification for the service, and as a result it becomes a variation to contract. Some companies have found out too late that they have mistakenly outsourced core services.

Meeting the customers   7.25

In the facilities context there are potential problems with outsourcing services that bring the contractor face to face with the customers of the service. Kotler and Bloom define service as:[2]

> 'any activity of benefit that one party can offer to another that is essentially intangible and does not result in ownership of anything. Its production may or may not be tied to a physical product.'

Services are performances not objects, and staff therefore need to be trained to give the correct performance for a variety of audiences. Contract staff need to be proficient in customer care and able to handle difficult situations as they arise.

Service specification   7.26

A lot of the early attempts at outsourcing failed due to poor specification. Often specifications were ill-prepared and incomplete, resulting in post-contract variations and escalating costs, or alternatively specifications were so detailed and complicated that it scared contractors off. There has been a shift away from detailed input specifications that are said to limit or stifle innovation towards output specifications that are less prescriptive and focus on the required service output.

Contract relationship   7.27

Often organisations have found out too late that they have exported valuable knowledge and expertise, which is difficult to place a price on and even more difficult to replace once it has been lost. That expertise and knowledge represents power and now it sits with the contract provider.

This shift of power is often exploited in the contract scenario in order to add leverage to decisions relating to extending the contract. The contractor will assess the competence of the informed client or the contracts manager during the mobilisation stage of the contract. If they know more about the outsourced service than the client, and if the knowledge and expertise has been transferred to the contractor as a result of outsourcing, then the contractor is placed in a very powerful position. This power shift may in itself be a spur to in-source the service and develop expertise, particularly if it is considered to be in an area of core activity. A decision to in-source based on this scenario will often be difficult, time-consuming and have high switching costs – but it is not impossible to achieve.

Supplier leverage   7.28

Supplier leverage can be demonstrated in a number of ways such as:

- price hikes;

- withholding access to new technology; and

- a reduction in the quality of work produced.

Lonsdale and Cox summarise the factors which lead to supplier leverage as follows:[3]

- **Poor contracting** – issues that are known within the firm are omitted from the contract. Either inappropriate personnel are assigned to the task of closing the deal, or the personnel concerned have inappropriate priorities.

- **Limited supply market options** – the firm chooses to outsource despite there being a limited number of supply options available to it.

- **High asset specificity** – because of the highly specific nature of the investment a firm makes in an outsourcing relationship, there is an effective absence of competition at the end of the contract period.

- **Uncertainty** – in situations where a firm has made highly specific investments, it will be even more vulnerable to supplier leverage if the nature of transaction between the buyer and the supplier is characterised by uncertainty. Uncertainty will lead to an incomplete contract, which will in time give the supplier the opportunity to charge excess fees.

When things go wrong   7.29

If outsourcing has failed to deliver, for whatever reason, it is important to revisit and dissect the circumstances and reasoning behind the original decision to outsource, and establish exactly why the process did not work, before making a kneejerk decision to in-source or revisit the market. Establish the current position before launching into a potential solution. It is essential that the way forward dovetails with both the facilities and the host organisation's strategy.

Analysis   7.30

Factors to consider when analysing the original decision are:

- In-house versus outsourced supply – re-visit the original decision to outsource.

174

- Core or non-core activity – does the service represent core activity?

- Service specification and contract – was the specification robust, relevant and kept up to date with requirements? Was there a contract in place?

- What benefits were perceived and what benefits were received?

- Contract management and performance monitoring – how effectively was the service monitored against the specification?

- Organisational change – people, process, and workplace.

- Contract relationship – power and leverage.

Service delivery   7.31

There are no off-the-peg solutions to the provision of FM. The portfolio of services and the range of options relating to the various combinations of service delivery have sparked discussion and debate over their respective merits.

Options include:

- In-house versus contract service provision, as discussed earlier in the chapter.

- Single-service or single-source contracts versus multi-service contract clusters, or total FM (TFM) contracts where one contractor manages and controls the entire facilities portfolio.

The risk here centres on economy of scale and knowledge within the organisation. Is it best to procure and manage a number of small and potentially quite demanding single-service contracts for a range of services, or to go for the one-stop shop approach? Each organisation needs to consider whether it has the time and expertise to manage single contracts and what the benefits of TFM might be to them.

The ultimate decision on the approach to take will depend on the organisation's unique requirements. One size does not fit all.

Changing fashions   7.32

Each approach will have risk attached to it, and advantages and disadvantages that need to be fully considered. The late 1980s and early 1990s were the era of the changing organisation, where 'out' was in, organisational hierarchy and management structures were flat and the customer was king. The traditional model of the organisation as it previously existed has been remodelled – its hierarchy and structure have been pulled apart, re-shaped and re-assembled, thus ensuring each component part is necessary and required and adds value to the delivered product or service.

Seamless service delivery   7.33

There has been a steady move away from the traditional methods of service delivery that in the past served to protect and support the practice of operating within controlled trade demarcation boundaries. These boundaries or service interface points between trade groups, staff groups, and contractors are steadily being eroded as service providers strive for the seamless approach to service delivery. It is in this remodelling that one of the key benefits of the facilities approach lies. Stripping out the inflexible barriers of demarcation can allow true innovation in how services are provided, and with this approach inefficiency can be eliminated.

Individuals can have more rewarding and more satisfying jobs that provide interest, flexibility and a degree of staff empowerment. True success in this approach rests in effective training, and clarity in the definition of role boundaries. The risks associated with multi-skilling and generic working need to be fully considered and comprehensive training, support and orientation provided to ensure that services are delivered in a safe and appropriate manner.

Obviously some factors, such as a change in statutory compliance requirements, will force strategic priority to be reconsidered. Once a strategy has been developed and objectives set it does not mean that a blinkered view must be taken.

Estates and facilities management in PFI   7.34

The NHS Plan (see **KEY REFERENCES, APPENDIX 1**) outlines a target for the NHS to deliver 100 new hospitals by 2010. There is also a drive to provide treatment centres, walk in centres and brand new GP surgeries and minor injuries units. The vast majority of the capital required to service this ambitious building programme will come from the private sector through PFI/PPP (Private Finance Initiative/Public Private Partnerships or NHS LIFT (Local Improvement Finance Trust) projects. This means that in the near future a significant part of the NHS Estate will be owned and operated by the private sector. PFI/PPP schemes are typically 25–35 years in duration. The NHS will continue to provide services within and from these premises and the patient environment and patient journeys will be greatly improved as a result. Risk transfer and value for money needs to be effectively demonstrated before a scheme is approved and authorised to proceed to the construction phase. Typically the risk of design, construction and operation are transferred to the PFI/PPP provider. During construction any cost or time overrun is at the contractor's risk. Risk transfer is further covered in **CHAPTER 3: MANAGING ORGANISATIONAL CHANGE**.

A typical PFI consortium will consist of a finance company (Funder), a constructor and a FM service provider. There are real benefits in bringing in the FM operators at an early stage to influence design and layout, as they will potentially be providing services in the building for the next 25–35 years so they need to influence material selection, design out maintenance, consider the front of house/back of house flows and logistic arrangements etc. In some deals the

PFI/PPP consortium take the risk on energy and utilities so it is essential that they select and manage systems and plant effectively.

These are long-term income streams and as mentioned earlier many FM providers are sinking equity into these deals. The funders (banks) are keen to ensure that the asset (hospital etc) remains serviceable and available in order to avoid financial penalty applied through the payment mechanism. Design therefore takes into account resilience of plant, infrastructure, staffing and planned redundancy of plant in order to ensure 100% availability. These new buildings are also maintained in strict accordance with an agreed lifecycle and maintenance plan in order to keep the building to condition B (safe and serviceable) unlike traditional NHS maintenance budgets which can be targets of cost reduction and efficiency savings, often at the expense of planned maintenance and recommended plant replacement frequencies. The banks engage the services of external technical advisors to ensure that maintenance and lifecycle plans are followed. A demonstration of this diligence could be the annual or six-monthly black start (total mains power drop out test and generator start up), although many hospital sites in the UK do not carry out this type of test.

In theory the building and its services will be maintained and refreshed during the life of the contract so that at the end of the concession the building is still in a Cat B condition prior to handover to the trust. It would therefore appear that PFI reduces the physical environment risk and manages an effective risk register.

The concession agreement and payment mechanism by which the Trust pay the PFI consortium for the building and the services they provide will state contractually that the PFI provider are to provide a safe and compliant site (statutory compliant) and that safe systems of work must be followed at all times, supported by risk assessments, PPE and training etc. If through trust or independent monitoring or audit, non-compliance, poor performance or health and Safety breaches are discovered, an award of penalty points (which could lead to the service provider being replaced) and high financial penalties can be applied.

On the face of it PFI/PPP reduces and manages significant risk with respect to the physical environment. Whilst this may be true in part, it must be noted that PFI is still in its infancy in healthcare. To date there are 15 first wave schemes that are fully operational, twelve financially closed (signed contracts) with work started on site and a further 36 major prioritised schemes with work at various stages. There is growing experience and standardisation with respect to procurement, scheme selection/evaluation, and construction/post project evaluation. However lessons are being learned in real time with respect to the operational delivery of PFI – making the contracts work. Many PFI constructors and service providers are new to healthcare design, construction and operation, although they have successful track records in other sectors. They too are learning lessons as they progress and it is essential that these lessons are shared from scheme to scheme. A key risk is managing the interface points of service delivery and managing variations to contract for space and services to support the changing healthcare requirements that will emerge in the future. Even though the trust does not own or operate all of the services it still has a duty of care.

A number of first wave schemes are looking to refinance their original deals. Now that the buildings/hospitals have been built the risk profile of the deals (particularly the first wave deals where uncertainty regarding the PFI process equalled risk which in turn lead to additional cost in order to mitigate the risk) have changed. Both the trust and the PFI provider share in the benefit of refinancing.

Facilities operational risk 7.35

A number of the statutory issues relating to FM services concern services and service infrastructure, which are often described as behind-the-scenes services.

These issues include:

- facilities risk management;

- pressure regulations;

- good practice in equipment maintenance;

- risk assessment for home workers;

- fire safety;

- electricity at work;

- security of staff and assets; and

- training and development.

These topics will be dealt with in turn below.

Facilities risk management

Health and safety legislation 7.36

Both employers and employees have a legal responsibility with respect to health and safety. It is essential that facilities managers, either in-house or outsourced, understand health and safety legislation and their duty of care, and put systems in place to comply with the legislation. It is vital that all facilities contractors are aware of the risks associated with their contracted place of work and of their own legal duties.

It is also essential that the facilities manager is satisfied that contractors comply with health and safety legislation and supporting guidance, and have conducted risk assessments (SEE CHAPTER 6). Routine monitoring of health and safety systems and procedures is recommended, and a compliance clause with respect to health and safety must be drafted into any specification or service level agreement (SLA). Good health and safety awareness and practice is a critical success factor for any organisation.

Health and safety legislation confers specific duties on employers, those in control of premises and employees to ensure health and safety at work. There are specific requirements for risk assessment. Risk assessments have to be robust, comprehensive, appropriate and kept up to date. Where there are five or more employees, significant findings of this assessment have to be recorded, and employers must draw up a health and safety policy statement and bring it to employees' attention. The requirement for a policy and risk assessment is fully explored in **CHAPTER 6**.

Risk assessment systems 7.37

There is an element of risk in all activities. Risk assessment is designed to identify high-risk activities and to ensure that safe systems of work are designed and adopted in order to minimise the risk. Each year about 1.1 million employees suffer workplace injury. This injury rate results in the loss of an estimated 30 million working days at a cost of £900 million a year to industry. Add to this extra costs to social security and the health service, and the loss of income by the victims, and the estimated overall total cost comes between £10–£15 billion per year.[4] Properly conducted risk assessment should reduce the likelihood of workplace injury and ill-health.

There are a number of paper-based and software systems designed to assist in the risk assessment process. Key areas to consider when conducting a workplace risk assessment relating to a task or activity include:

- air quality and temperature, water systems, pressure systems;

- electricity, fire, noise, asbestos and hazardous substances;

- lighting, trailing leads, glass openings, doors and gates, and mobile work equipment;

- staff facilities, personal protective equipment, visual display units and manual handling;

- first aid, sanitation and washing facilities; and

- disability access.

Pressure Regulations 7.38

The main Regulations covering pressure systems and pressure equipment are the *Pressure Equipment Regulations 1999 (SI 1999/2001)* and the *Pressure System Safety Regulations 2000 (SI 2000/128)*. The failure of operational pressure equipment or pressure systems – resulting in the uncontrolled release of pressurised agents – could kill or seriously injure people nearby and cause considerable damage to property.

Typical pressure systems 7.39

In a healthcare setting, examples of typical pressure systems and equipment are as follows:

- pipework and associated hoses;
- autoclaves and pressure cookers;
- steam systems, including steam traps or filters, and valves;
- boilers;
- compressed air systems; and
- pressure gauges and indicators.

The main reasons for pressure system failures are:

- poor installation, design and equipment specification;
- poor maintenance and system repair;
- unsafe work systems; and
- operator error, poor supervision and training.

Failure of a pressure system can cause the following:

- fire – due to the uncontrolled release of chemical, whether liquid or gas;
- impact from flying debris or equipment parts, or blast impact; and
- contact with released contents of the pressure system – steam or gas.

Avoiding pressure system failure 7.40

A series of measures can be put into place in order to reduce the risk of pressure system or equipment failure. These are:

- Design the system and install it in accordance with appropriate standards, specifications, guidance and Regulations.
- Ensure that safety devices are installed.
- Regularly inspect the system/equipment and maintain it at the required frequency – using suitable materials and spares.
- Develop and adopt a safe system of work.
- Provide appropriate training on the system for all relevant staff.
- Develop operating procedures and clear working instructions and ensure that they are kept updated. The operating instructions should include the operating condition of the product under pressure (for example, gas) and instructions for dealing with emergency conditions.
- If the system is extended or altered ensure that the training, maintenance procedures, spares and operating instructions and plans are updated to reflect the changes and the requirements and condition of the changed system.

Examination of pressure systems 7.41

A written scheme of examination drawn up by a competent person is required for all pressure systems, except those classified as exempt in *Schedule 1* of the *Pressure Systems Safety Regulations 2000 (SI 2000/128)*. Pressure systems must not be used without having a written scheme of examination. The written scheme must cover all pipework, vessels and protective devices.

Good practice in equipment maintenance 7.42

In many organisations the maintenance equipment and the physical environment forms the backbone to the facilities remit – perhaps because many facilities managers have a building or engineering background. Maintenance will undoubtedly form a major part of any SLA or contract when it is included in the facilities remit, but FM is not about being an expert in all areas or professional disciplines.

Therefore, maintenance does not necessarily have to be managed or controlled by an estates professional. In many organisations the facilities team may be very lean and expert advice is bought in as and when required. This can also apply to estates consultancy, as in some organisations, the entire range of estate-related services has been outsourced to the contract sector.

It is perfectly feasible for a personnel, human resources or facilities manager with a catering background to have responsibility for site maintenance within their total facilities remit. There is a mystique surrounding the management of maintenance that it is riddled with risk and statutory obligation to such an extent that it 'must' be managed by estate professionals.

Statutory obligation and risk management do indeed form key components in the safe and effective management of estate and property; however, the key is to ensure sound back-up and advice on maintenance, either from within the FM team or from an independent consultant on a retainer.

Outsourcing maintenance 7.43

It is preferable to keep the advisory role separate from the maintenance contract, as a sharp operator will identify areas of weakness and vulnerability and could exploit them. However, it may be equally desirable to outsource the provision and management of maintenance to a contractor completely – in which case the facilities manager needs to identify the budget and the specification and leave the delivery and innovation to them. In this scenario, agreement on the specification and monitoring systems is vital.

The specification must be comprehensive and include plant asset lists, life cycle costing definitions, schedules of rates for repair works, cost threshold levels, and so on. The final decision will be unique to each organisation. The method of service delivery will greatly depend on the size of the organisation, the scale of the FM function and economy of scale with respect to contract bundling of services.

Types of maintenance   7.44

This section will briefly outline the management of planned and unplanned maintenance with a view to minimising risk relating to maintenance and operations.

The definitions of various types of maintenance, taken from British Standards, are as follows:

- **Maintenance** – the combination of all technical and associated administrative actions intended to retain an item in, or restore it to, a state in which it can perform its required function (BS 3811: 1984).

- **Maintenance programme** – a time-based plan allocating specific maintenance tasks to specific periods (BS 3811: 1984).

- **Breakdown maintenance** – the operation of restoring an item to a state in which it can fulfil its original function after a failure in its performance (BS 8210: 1986).

- **Corrective maintenance** – the maintenance carried out after a failure has occurred and intended to restore an item to a state in which it can perform its required function (BS 3811: 1984).

- **Emergency maintenance** – the maintenance which it is necessary to put in hand immediately to avoid serious consequences (BS 3811: 1984).

- **Repair** – restoration of an item to an acceptable condition by the renewal, replacement or mending of worn, damaged or decayed parts (BS 8210: 1986).

- **Remedial work** – redesign and work necessary to restore the integrity of a construction to a standard that will allow the performance of its original function (BS 8210: 1986).

- **Planned maintenance** – maintenance organised and carried out with forethought, control and the use of records, to a predetermined plan based on the results of previous condition surveys.

- **Condition-based maintenance** – preventative maintenance initiated as a result of knowledge of an item's condition gained from routine or continuous monitoring (BS 3811: 1984).

- **Preventative maintenance** – maintenance carried out at predetermined intervals, or corresponding to prescribed criteria, and intended to reduce the probability of failure or performance degradation of an item (BS 3811: 1984).

The above list could be divided into two groups – planned (programmed) maintenance and unplanned (response) maintenance. This brief outline is intended to define these two types of maintenance and to highlight the need to offset the peaks and troughs of unplanned maintenance with planned work. In this way responsiveness to the unknown and unplanned can be balanced with statutory compliance, service requirements and frequencies.

Planned and unplanned maintenance   7.45

Unplanned maintenance can be broken down into a further two categories:

- normal response; and
- emergency response.

Planned maintenance can similarly be broken down into:

- preventative; and
- cyclical.

Service delivery   7.46

Critical systems (such as nurse call, power supplies, or a renal water treatment plant) and their associated service response and rectification times will need to be outlined in the SLA for each location. The helpdesk (see below) can be utilised to generate data that relates to requests for maintenance and repair of these systems, and this data enables a comparison between actual (time from request to repair) and stated SLA response and rectification. This approach will highlight performance, and areas where resources should be targeted in order to maximise the availability of labour, spares and consumables.

Maintenance systems operated as part of a helpdesk or computer-aided facilities management (CAFM) system usually work on a job ticket or docket system. Dockets or requests are issued to contractors or trades people. These will include details of the location, a description of the fault and an agreed response time. Some also include an allowance for or estimate of the time required to complete the repair. Planned maintenance dockets may have the service routine printed on the docket to aid the tradesman. The request or docket will also include a cost code used to log all labour costs and spares or consumables used during repair or maintenance. Goods will generally only be issued against a request or docket and they are immediately coded against the cost code for recharging purposes.

Effective logging   7.47

Some contracts or SLAs operate against a schedule of agreed rates (costs per hour) for breakdown maintenance with spares used in repairs charged extra to contract. In theory all consumables used during a planned service should have been quantified and included in the contract or SLA. Some of the more sophisticated maintenance software systems have bar codes printed onto the dockets, to enable the completed job requests and supplies requisitions to be scanned straight into the computer in order to log labour hours and materials, thereby cutting down on the amount of manual data entry required. It is vital that all planned requests or job dockets are completed and fed back into the system in order to collect costs, response times, materials used and status of repair.

The system can also be used to log plant history and maintenance frequency – this is important for statutory maintenance tests for pressure vessels or electrical installations. By following this type of approach to maintenance, it will ensure that as far as possible systems and equipment are maintained in accordance with manufacturers' recommendations and that all maintenance tasks are recorded along with spares used and the details of the person carrying out the task. This provides a full service history. It is also important to log when planned routines have been rescheduled or pulled forward – perhaps to take advantage of downtime or a shutdown – to ensure that the number of planned maintenance visits stated in the specification or the SLA are delivered.

Planned preventative maintenance   7.48

Planned preventative maintenance (PPM) is usually programmed on a cyclical basis. For example, a heating system will need to be maintained under PPM at the following frequencies:

- weekly;
- six-weekly;
- quarterly;
- half-yearly; and
- yearly.

A maintenance routine will be drawn up that takes into account the manufacturer's service requirements, replacement frequency and any local implications. A series of tasks or checks will be scheduled against the PPM frequencies. Six-weekly tasks include the weekly tasks plus some additional checks or service requirements; quarterly tasks include the six-weekly tasks, and so on.

Planning ahead   7.49

In order to plan workload and manpower resources, all of the PPM maintenance frequencies need to be entered into the maintenance program or work planner. The program will look at all of the site's PPM tasks over a year and highlight where there is a clash of routines – perhaps 20 quarterly routines have been programmed for the same week, which it would not be possible to resource.

Most maintenance programs have a feature that allows workload to be planned over a given period to achieve best fit with available resources plus an allowed percentage for unplanned response. For example, a maintenance department could base its operations on a ratio of 70% PPM to 30% unplanned or repair work. If this were the case, an estimate of the total PPM hours required for the stated workload over the year could be used to establish the level of manpower or resources required to service the specification or SLA, with a buffer of generic working to ensure 100% utilisation of the labour pool in a productive manner. While there is some flexibility to offset peaks and troughs of demand and planned/unplanned workload, some maintenance tasks are statutory (equipment must be inspected and results documented at stated frequencies) and therefore must be completed at the defined PPM frequencies. In addition, maintenance of large boiler plant, pressure vessels and lifts will have an insurance implication and will need to be inspected during maintenance by an appropriate insurance engineer.

Effective maintenance   7.50

The following steps are essential in order to effectively manage maintenance:

- Identify and comply with any statutory obligations.

- Identify and assess all risks.

- Produce a detailed asset register of all plant and equipment.

- Produce a comprehensive specification (input or output).

- Develop safe systems of work based on risk assessments of all tasks.

- Identify key components or items of equipment vital to business continuity and prioritise maintenance tasks/spares.

- Develop a PPM schedule for key items of plant and equipment.

- Provide appropriate training and support for maintenance staff.

- Record and document maintenance performance and test results.

- Agree a process and a specification for a helpdesk or work requisitioning/ scheduling system.

- Agree a schedule of rates for unplanned maintenance.

- Communicate with other parts of the organisation.

Note that capital investment appraisal and life cycle costing are not included in the above list. It is assumed that the elements of life cycle costing – including purchase, installation, commissioning, operation, spares, consumables and disposal – have all been fully considered prior to asset purchase as part of the investment appraisal. Therefore planned maintenance costs and training or familiarisation have been budgeted for before the asset is put to use and requires maintenance support.

Risk assessment for homeworkers   7.51

With the ready availability of reliable and relatively inexpensive data and telecommunication technology, more and more staff are choosing to work from home if their work patterns and duties allow it. The *Workplace (Health, Safety and Welfare) Regulations 1992 (SI 1992/3004)* do not cover the home although an employer's duty of care to protect the health and safety of their employees still applies regardless of where they work.

The *Management of Health and Safety at Work Regulations 1999 (SI 1999/3242)* place a requirement on employers to carry out a risk assessment of the work activities carried out by homeworkers, identifying the hazards relating to the home-working activities.

Most responsible employers will either carry out a home-based workplace risk assessment or will have an assessment audit tool that home-based employees can complete themselves. The assessment should cover a range of standard items such as:

*   lighting;
*   electrical power and socket requirements;
*   storage space, the working environment and ergonomics;
*   security;
*   display screen equipment; and
*   fire safety.

Fire precautions and risk assessment   7.52

The legal requirements with regard to safety from fire where people are employed to work are, in the main, one or both of two pieces of legislation:

*   The *Fire Precautions Act 1971*.
*   The *Fire Precautions (Workplace) Regulations 1997 (SI 1997/1840)*.

Guidance   7.53

Specific guidance on fire engineering in hospitals and healthcare establishments is available from the suite of 17 documents that make up *Firecode*.[5] Each of the documents focuses on specific applications relating to fire. Three of the main documents are:

*   Health Technical Memorandum (HTM) 81 – Fire precautions in new hospitals.

- HTM 85 – Fire precautions in existing hospitals.

- HTM 86 – Fire risk assessment in hospitals.

The *Building Regulations 1991 (SI 1991/2768) (Approved Document B)* detail the fire safety measures required in new buildings and buildings which are to be extended or structurally altered.

A specific safety standard is also included in controls assurance (see **KEY REFERENCES, APPENDIX** 1), which sets out a number of fire safety criteria by which to measure fire safety performance. The criteria mirror both mandatory and statutory obligations along with best practice guidance.

Health Service Circular   7.54

Health Service Circular 1999/191[6] set out the ministerial priorities with respect to fire engineering in healthcare establishments. The circular states that:

- No patient area is to be in an unsafe condition – that is, no areas to remain in estate code condition D – by 31 March 2001, or an outline business case to support improvement is to be in place to support this initiative.

- Backlog work is to be eradicated by 31 March 2003.

This circular has served as a focus for fire safety improvement and provides a non-negotiable end point for eradication of the fire safety backlog by early 2003.

Fire engineering and design   7.55

HTM 81 provides guidance relating to fire engineering and design in new hospital buildings and takes into account important fire issues such as escape, evacuation, and compartmentation – that is, control of the spread of fire. It is vital that fire engineering is considered at the design stage. The local fire service and the planning authority will take particular interest in applications relating to the design and upgrade of healthcare establishments.

HTM 85 provides guidance on similar issues to *HTM 81*, but is focused on upgrade, retrofit and overcoming inadequacy in the fire engineering elements of design components of existing buildings.

Annual fire risk assessment   7.56

An annual fire risk assessment must be carried out in all areas of a hospital.

The assessment should cover the following areas, as required by *HTM 86*:

- **Hazards** – ignition sources such as smoking, arson, equipment, and work processes. This will identify if the trust has a no-smoking policy, localised risks of arson, and location and storage of potentially hazardous equipment such as gas bottles. It will also highlight potentially hazardous work practices carried out in the locality, such as welding.

- **Combustible materials and surface finishes** – this covers the presence of significant potential fire load and expanses of varnished wood panelling, furniture, and fabrics.

- **Precautions** – fire prevention measures, fire barriers, and smoke dampers.

- **Communications** – alarm and detection systems, and zone plans.

- **Means of escape** – fire exits, escape routes and signage.

- **Containment** – structural elements, fire compartmentation and fire protection to hazard areas.

- **Extinguishment** – availability and suitability of fire-fighting equipment.

All of the above are scored as being either:

1. High standard.

2. Acceptable risk/hazard or *HTM 85* standard.

3. High risk/hazard.

4. Very high risk/hazard.

5. Inadequate.

6. Unacceptable.

Balancing life risks, hazards and precautions 7.57

HTM 86 provides an approach to risk assessment based on balancing life risks, fire hazards and existing fire precautions. Regular fire risk assessment needs to be carried out and should not just focus on active and passive fire detection, but also identify local issues that may cause fire problems, such as clutter in fire escape routes, the risk of arson, storage of combustible materials or medical gas cylinders.

Some healthcare buildings may require fire certificates. This requirement will be dependent, for example, on the design and layout of the building, the number of staff in the building and the work process taking place in the building. Discussion should take place with the local fire authority to determine which buildings they consider should have fire certificates. Staff should be made aware of the fire-related risks pertinent to the area that they work in. This awareness should cover passive and active fire detection, fire-fighting equipment location and its appropriate use, and fire signage/escape route and evacuation procedures.

FPN 11 reducing unwanted fire signals in healthcare premises is a relatively new addition in 2003 and it is intended to be used in all healthcare premises in acute and primary care settings. Its aim is to limit the amount of false fire alarms caused for example by cookers, toasters and contractors working.

Electricity at work   7.58

Statistics indicate that there are about 1,000 accidents at work involving electric shock or burns each year that get reported to the HSE. Around 30 of these are fatal. Most of these fatalities arise from contact with overhead or underground power cables. There are basic but effective measures that can be adopted in order to control the risks relating to the use of electricity at work.

Main hazards   7.59

The main hazards are:

- contact with live parts causing burns and electric shock (mains voltage can kill);

- explosion or fire where electricity could be the potential source of ignition in explosive or flammable atmospheres; and

- electrical faults that could cause fires.

In order to reduce the risks associated with electricity, the risks must be identified by a full risk assessment. This identifies the hazards, evaluates the risk arising from the hazards and identifies who might be harmed as a result and how. The risks associated with the use of electricity at work are amplified when electricity is used in surroundings, which are:

- **outdoors** – perhaps outside of the electrical zone of protection;

- **wet** – which under certain circumstances could cause unsuitable equipment to become live; and

- **confined or cramped** – particularly when working in tanks, bins or silos involving close proximity to large surface areas of earthed metalwork which make it difficult to avoid shock.

Reducing risks   7.60

Risk associated with electricity can be reduced by:

- **Reducing the voltage** – such as portable power tools running at 110 volts, temporary lighting operating at a reduced voltage or in some circumstances the use of battery powered tools or air/hand powered tools.

- **Maintenance and inspection** – it is essential to ensure that existing electrical installations are safe and are regularly maintained so as to keep them in a safe condition.

- **Conforming to standards** – new electrical installations should be designed in accordance with the Institution of Electrical Engineers wiring regulations and installed to a suitable standard such as *BS 7671* –

Requirements for electrical installations and associated guidance notes. This standard does not have statutory power but provides a useful indication of good industrial practice in meeting the *Electricity at Work Regulations 1989 (SI 1989/635).*

- **Testing** – electrical installation and testing is now being linked to a new specific section of the Building Regulations and this move will see a structured and formalised approach to regular testing of installations – carried out by specialist testing professionals. Installations should be regularly maintained and tested for safe operation. Testing should also include a visual inspection to identify damaged or fraying power leads, or overloaded power sockets. Fixed installations should be tested periodically by a competent person; records of these periodic tests are useful for plant history and for assessing the effectiveness of the installation.

- **Provision of safety devices** – it is vital that electrical circuits have adequate and effective protection afforded by circuit breakers, fuses, or residual circuit breakers. As electrical distribution systems are extended or adapted to meet current demand requirements, the type and rating of the circuit protection must be checked in order to ensure that the type of protection provided is still appropriate. It is also important to ensure that circuit overload and rating of the protection is correct, in order to protect the installation and the users, and that circuit discrimination is maintained. The protection device closest to the fault should operate first.

- **Suitable equipment** – equipment must be suitable for the environment in which it will be used and must be maintained regularly in order to ensure that it is safe and functioning correctly. It is good practice to keep a list of all electrical equipment, portable tools and appliances and record test results.

- **Safe working systems** – ensure that people who are working with electricity are competent to do so. Work on or near exposed live parts must not be allowed unless it is absolutely unavoidable and suitable precautions have been taken to prevent injury, both to the workers and to anyone else who may be in the area. Thorough risk assessment must be undertaken and documented outlining why it has been assessed as unavoidable to work on or near to exposed live parts.

Security of staff and assets   7.61

Security of staff and assets is everyone's responsibility, but there is very little in the way of legislative requirement to provide security. The only statutory requirements to take security measures are either:

- general duties to provide a safe and healthy place of work for employees; and

- specific requirements where there are issues of national patient security or where explosives or dangerous substances are being stored.

There may also be contractual responsibilities requiring employers to protect people and assets. Where equipment is required to maintain the safety of employees, such as a closed-circuit television (CCTV) system for staff working in a potentially vulnerable location, this is covered under the *Provision and Use of Work Equipment Regulations 1998 (SI 1998/2306)*. It should be noted that the *Data Protection Act 1998* also contains specific requirements relating to the management of CCTV systems. Employers may wish to impose a confidentiality agreement as part of the employment contract in healthcare establishments.

Security needs to be considered as part of a wider approach to risk management, which addresses risks to people, property and the business. Most healthcare establishments have systems in place to cover bomb threats, suspect packages, business continuity, and fraud (as discussed in **CHAPTER 8**) and this demonstrates that security-related risks have been assessed in part. However, security management in healthcare establishments is a growing area of risk that needs to have focus and high visibility.

Zero tolerance 7.62

The NHS has taken a hard-line, zero tolerance approach to crime and violence in hospitals, where staff can be subjected to physical or verbal abuse from patients, their families and the public. This is no longer generally tolerated and must not be accepted as part of the day-to-day consequence of providing healthcare. However it is not just those working in accident and emergency or staff at the acute end that are subject to abuse – often reception staff and staff working in areas with public interaction, such as outpatients, restaurants and portering, that face security problems. Violence and aggression in healthcare is also covered in **CHAPTER 6**.

The Health and Safety Executive (HSE) defines work-related violence as:

> 'Any incident in which a person is abused, threatened or assaulted in circumstances relating to their work'

This can include verbal abuse or threats as well as physical attacks. The HSE has recently commissioned research into the effectiveness of training in the management of violence and aggression in healthcare.

Risk assessment, training in defusing aggression or conflict resolution, physical barriers or secure design approaches and CCTV can minimise these risks. Many trusts have implemented sophisticated ID badge and access control systems to assist in security management in healthcare establishments; these systems can be used to manage staff, visitors and contractors. There is always a trade-off in hospitals between ease of access and the need for security, and this trade-off will impact in different ways at each site.

A local solution must be sought following a thorough risk assessment that looks at the building and the way it is used. Risk assessment should also identify lone working practices. An important aspect of the assessment is to to identify areas that may become a target for theft, such as cash handling offices, or areas where computers or attractive consumables are stored. A security strategy complete with operating policies and procedures relating to the risks identified will assist in the management of these risks, and will aid communication with staff.

Training and development 7.63

Training and development is an area that has been overlooked in the past with regard to facilities staff. All too often staff are unable to be released from their day-to-day operational duties, or cannot be covered by colleagues during training sessions. It is in the interests of both employer and employee to ensure that appropriate and timely training is given and received. Indeed given the frequency of new and updated statutory legislation and guidance, it is vital that staff are kept abreast of new requirements, guidance and techniques.

Recruitment and retention 7.64

A major risk facing many healthcare employers (particularly those in the South of England where unemployment is low and healthcare salaries are uncompetitive) is recruitment and ongoing retention. Employers need to be creative with the employment package on offer to attract and keep the right staff. Training should not therefore be limited to statutory updates or an annual fire lecture. Employment packages do not solely consist of pay – the opportunity for training and development may also be attractive to staff. The importance of professional development is dealt with in **CHAPTER 9**. The skills and competencies of each member of staff should be assessed, to inform a structured training and personal development plan. This should contain updates on health, safety and statutory issues.

What should training include? 7.65

Training can be provided initially during staff induction and orientation and basic fire safety training – looking at the location of fire exits, fire fighting equipment, and break glass points. General organisational policies such as infection control, clinical waste segregation, and security should also be provided. It is also beneficial to demonstrate to staff the sound of fire and other alarms. Basic lifting and handling training should be provided tailored to the activity that the employee carries out. Information regarding the control of substances hazardous to health and workplace risk assessments should also be explained to new starters so that they are made fully aware of risk in their workplace and of the procedures in place to identify and minimise those risks. Health and safety training requirements are more specifically discussed in **CHAPTER 6**.

Giving staff further responsibilities 7.66

Over time as staff become familiar and comfortable with the workplace they could be encouraged to take on responsibility for specific areas of risk management in their locality, such as becoming the local fire marshal, local health and safety representative, or the local back care trainer. Appropriate training will need to be provided to support these duties but this approach leads to broader awareness of specific and general aspects of risk management in the workplace, and encourages a sense of ownership for workplace health and safety.

At given periods, staff with specific technical training – such as the medical gas authorised person, high voltage/low voltage electricity authorised person, steriliser engineers, or catering staff – will need to have a refresher or update course. It is important that employers therefore treat staff training and development seriously and manage the process of delivery.

A methodical approach 7.67

This chapter has outlined the importance, scale and complexity of risk relating to the physical environment and the operational aspects of supporting healthcare delivery. It has been shown that due to the diverse nature of service delivery and premises, a proactive but methodical approach is required in order to identify and deal appropriately with risk in this dynamic environment.

Management of these risks needs to link into the strategic view of the organisation in order to identify and consider the impact of actions implemented to manage or reduce an area of risk. Facilities managers also need to be in a position to provide advice and guidance on the risks associated with changes to service delivery. Risk also needs to be effectively managed across the virtual organisation that makes up the facilities team – comprised of contractors, project workers, architects, outsourced service providers and PFI partners. The trust's authorised officer needs to be certain that contract partners have a robust grasp of risk management, consistent with the trust's overall approach to managing risk.

Concordat 7.68

At a strategic and national level, in 2003 a concordat was drawn up by the HSE and NHS Estates – designed to act as a framework to guide future working between the HSE and NHS Estates. Translating the roles and responsibilities of the two organizations into practical working arrangements. Hopefully this approach will ensure that policy, procedure and guidance are able to be implemented embedded into organisational culture in a seamless manner.

References

See also KEY REFERENCES, APPENDIX 1
1   Handy, C (1994) *The Empty Raincoat*, Hutchinson, London.
2   Kotler, P and Bloom, PM (1999) *Marketing Professional Services*, Free Press, New York, USA.
3   Lonsdale, C and Cox, A (1998) *Outsourcing: a business guide to risk management tools and techniques*, Boston, Earlsgate.

4   Unpublished research conducted by Trevor Payne.
5   *Firecode*, NHS Estates (tel: 0113 254 7299 or *www.nhsestates.gov.uk/property_ manage-ment/content/fire_code.html*).
6   Health Service Circular 1999/191 (*www.doh.gov.uk*).

HSE Guidance

Check the HSE website for the most up-to-date guidance at *www.hse.gov.uk* or call the HSE infoline on 08701 545500. HSE Information Services, Caerphilly Business Park, Caerphilly CF83 3GG.

HSE (1998) *Five steps to risk assessment*

HSE (1998) *Electrical safety and you*

HSE (1993) *Electricity at work – safe working practices*

HSE (1994) *Essentials of health and safety at work*

HSE (1994) HSG 107: *Maintaining portable and transportable electrical equipment*

HSE (1994) *Written Schemes of Examination*

Workplace (Health, Safety and Welfare) Regulations 1992. Approved Code of Practice and Guidance

British Standards

(1984) BS 3811: Glossary of Maintenance Management Terms, British Standards Institution, London (www.bsi-global.com).

(1986) BS 8210: Guide to Building Maintenance Management.

(1992) BS 7671: Requirements for electrical installations and IEE wiring regulations: guidance notes.

Further reading

Barret, P (ed.) (1996) *Facilities Management: Towards Best Practice*, Blackwell Science, Oxford.

British Institute of Facilities Management (1999) *Survey of facilities managers' responsibilities*, BIFM, Saffron Walden. (*www.bifm.org.uk*)

NHS Estates (1996) *Re-engineering the Facilities Management Service*, Health Facilities Note 16.

Payne, T (2000) *Facilities Management – a strategy for success*, Chandos Publishing, Oxford.

Web links

www.hmso.gov.uk

www.hse.gov.uk/campaigns/asbestos

NHS Zero Tolerance Campaign (www.nhs.uk/zerotolerance/intro.htm)

Chapter 8
Service Continuity Management

This chapter covers:

- The definition of service continuity management.
- The nature of disasters in healthcare.
- The impact of service interruption.
- Developing service continuity plans.
- Implementation of service continuity plans.
- Resources service continuity management.
- Strategic benefits.

Introduction   8.1

Within risk management circles, the concept of business continuity management is not new and is applied with varying degrees of rigour in commerce and industry. In the service sector, however, the use of the term 'business continuity' does not sit comfortably with many professionals. The services they provide are not for profit, and are normally delivered in accordance with best practice and value for money. Accordingly, the term 'service continuity' tends to be used.

Either term encapsulates the philosophy of establishing a way of working that will ensure service delivery regardless of a major interruption to normal activity. Ideally, a plan of action should exist which will ensure seamless recovery from a disaster.

History and background

Disaster recovery   8.2

Since the introduction of the computer age, managers have recognised the importance of their stored data and have ensured against the instability of their machines and potential corruption of data by creating secondary copies and, if wise, storing the data off site. This process became known as disaster recovery or DR. The technique became familiar to IT professionals but remained little understood by general management.

Business recovery 8.3

With the passage of time and the introduction of distributed systems via servers, networks, and personal computers, information systems are now an integral support function to organisations, rather than separate systems in their own right. Managers began to consider investing in broader disaster recovery contingency plans. However, they soon realised that if a disaster happened – say, a major fire in a production area – the fact that the computer could be restored while the work accommodation for staff could not, seemed a little like putting the cart before the horse. From this developed the term 'business recovery' which involves not just the computer systems but importantly the organisational facilities, processes and human resources interaction.

Maintaining business as usual 8.4

Nowadays the speed of service delivery has increased and the concept of business recovery has been found in practice to be too little too late. It is not sufficient to simply recover from a disaster, since during the downtime customers may have lost patience and moved their business to a competitor. Instead, it is now necessary to examine how to maintain business as usual. For this new situation, the term 'business continuity' is used. This incorporates the strategic vision of an organisation while maintaining its customer service.

In the service and healthcare sector, the prospect of clients moving to a competitor does not exist in quite the same way as in commercial organisations, although doubtless any major impact to service delivery at a specific establishment may influence referral patterns, the purchase of services and patient outcomes. The public are increasingly less tolerant of service delays or interruption and measure an organisation's reputation and its public face by how well the organisation manages its continuous operation. An added complication to maintaining business as usual relates to PPI hospitals which are owned and operated by an external 'consortium'. In such hospitals the development of contingency plans will need to involve many more players.

The need to have contingency plans in place has been recognised for some time in larger hospitals, and many initiatives have been tried and tested. It is possible to develop simple but effective service continuity plans. The basis for successful planning is executive sponsorship and adoption of a top–down approach. This means planning for prioritised impact mitigation, rather than for every possible eventuality.

What is service continuity management?   8.5

The use of the phrase 'service continuity management' is deliberate. It is a management process and it needs to be championed from the top of an organisation. Often the term continuity planning is used, but this is only one part of the process of managing the service continuity of the organisation. Circumstances, procedures and staff changes mean that the process must be ongoing, with a regular schedule of review and update. Essentially, management must strive for a constant state of preparedness at all levels.

For service continuity management to be effective, a strategic decision must be made at executive level to put in place an action plan. This must be robust and comprehensive enough to ensure the continuity of core services even in the event of a major incident. It is not just about putting a plan in place as part of a new initiative; it must be recognised as part of the risk management process of ongoing mitigation and preparedness. It must be seen as a change to 'the way things are done round here.'

Defining a 'major incident'   8.6

Part of the plan-building process requires the term 'major incident' to be defined. Such a definition can be based upon the existing definition contained within the major incident plan (MIP) of larger hospitals for external incidents, such as civil emergencies or road traffic accidents. The service continuity plan is, however, concerned with internal incidents. These incidents may or may not be equal in size to the external incident addressed by the MIP, but they do have very real impacts upon the organisation in terms of resolving the hazard or problem and managing the issues and implications arising from the incident. To be successful, it is necessary to prioritise and categorise activities within the organisation and determine each function's tolerance to interruption, in terms of:

- impact on interdependencies up-stream (who supplies us) and down-stream (who critically depends on us);

- scale, that is the minimum post-loss resource requirements for staff, accommodation, equipment, networks and communications; and

- duration (hours, days, weeks or longer).

Usually a major internal incident can be defined in terms of:

- preventing more than one function from continuing with its normal operations as a result of a genuine threat to life, facilities, utilities, and equipment; and

- falling outside the scope of normal management arrangements, with the potential to materially affect the activities or reputation of the organisation.

Threats to service continuity   8.7

There are many threats impacting on a healthcare organisation's ability to deliver its services and serve the community. These can have an impact on both clinical and non-clinical areas (see box).

Potential threats

- Fire or explosion affecting a department or centralised energy centre.

- Severe weather leading to flooding or burst pipes.

- Theft of care equipment.

- Hacking leading to breaches of data protection legislation and security of patient records.

- Supply chain failure in domestic or hotel services.

- IT system failure blocking access to patient administration systems.

- Sub-standard performance in hygiene, catering, or clinical care.

- Infrastructure interruption, such as loss of utilities, medical gas supply or voice and data communication.

All healthcare providers whether multi or single sited would recognise a major fire as an expensive and inconvenient interruption to service delivery with the real potential to harm patients and staff. The impact is not determined by the cause, but rather the effect on the organisation's service delivery. For example, consider the loss, by fire, to a hospital, of four medical wards versus loss of the centralised laundry. Which has the larger impact? By contrast, the local ambulance station providing a 24-hour service to a number of client trusts would find it almost impossible to operate if the manufacturer of its fleet recommended a recall on safety grounds.

So we see that the impact of a major incident varies from one organisation to another. The philosophy of service continuity management is geared towards reducing the impact of interruption to a specific service by restoring its critical functions, irrespective of the nature of the disaster.

Potential impact of incidents   8.8

For NHS organisations, potential impact equates to loss of service provision to any client group in the community. It is the standard of front-line services as judged by the public that sets the pace for continuity. Often, back-office support and management are not immediately critical.

Many organisations have failed to implement a service continuity culture simply by making a fundamental error – that is, misjudging what needs to be planned for.

Many organisations recognise the need to conduct risk assessments, and in the process anticipate a considerable range of potential eventualities. An immediate response to this is often to seek to develop a contingency arrangement for each and every risk. This is simply an impossible task, as in any organisation there are many interdependencies and possibilities. Much time and resource will be expended attempting to come up with practical solutions that avoid the creation of other problems. A tactical solution or fix must be matched by an equally robust strategic consideration of the issues arising from any proposed solution.

Inability to provide a service is the worst-case scenario and can be encapsulated in terms of loss of premises, systems, staff and equipment. This is what should be considered when planning. If the impact of an event is not as serious as this, an organisation will be able to continue to use those services that remain to best effect.

How incidents are managed, and are seen to be managed, can have a significant impact on an organisation's reputation and its ability to recover in the eyes of the community. A post-incident communication strategy is therefore a sensible measure.

The nature of disasters in healthcare   8.9

Some would argue that our working life is a constant series of crises or disasters – but this is not the case. It is the out-of-the-ordinary event that must be considered in service continuity planning.

Crises do not need to become disasters if they are managed correctly. Often in the healthcare sector, crisis communication is as important as crisis management. The news media will always pick up on a human story, such as:

- patient records found at the public refuse centre;
- body parts found on a landfill site;
- failure of management control over radiation doses for radiotherapy;
- collapse of a patient record archive and library system;
- failure of life support systems;
- newly installed kitchens failing to meet food hygiene requirements; or
- power failures in a newly built hospital.

Mercifully the application of fire regulations in hospitals has resulted in very few catastrophic incidents relating to fire, so it is more worthwhile to look at other risks.

Causes of disaster   8.10

Disaster stories in the healthcare sector tend to focus on the organisation's treatment of a group of individuals. The Department of Health's report *An*

Organisation with a Memory (see **KEY REFERENCES, APPENDIX 1**) states that incidents in trusts can be attributed to:

- 92% – lack of communication and systems.

- 8% – human error.

However, in reality most incidents are simply blamed on human error rather than recognising that the system might need to be reviewed. Systems should be in place to minimise the risk of error in human activity and in electro-mechanical devices.

If we consider near-misses or behaviour that could lead to a disaster, in light of the above, an example at a newly completed hospital with an adjacent energy centre proves the case in point (see box below).

We see in this example that a procedure not only needs to be documented, but also applied and enforced. A change in the cultural attitude to risk management is required. All parties in an organisation, whether public or private sector partners, must adopt an integrated approach. This is precisely the intended outcome from applying the standards in the NHS controls assurance programme (see **KEY REFERENCES, APPENDIX 1**).

Jamming the door

The energy centre is in a separate, secure compound area at a major hospital, with an emergency exit door giving direct access to the main street. Inside the building are all the controls and plant to provide the hospital with standby power generation, day-to-day heating, ventilation and air conditioning.

The safe operation of the centre is placed with a service contractor subject to the professional controls expected for such a facility, including swipe card access control. Employees of the service contractor were formerly NHS trust staff and have close relations with trust staff employed in hotel duties. For ease of access to local shops, non-authorised trust personnel had bypassed the access control system with cooperation from contracted operating staff. Using the energy centre as a short cut, they had jammed the final exit door ajar so as to make their way to and from the hospital, instead of using the main entrance and road management system, which would take longer.

This is not an isolated example but it highlights the potential for self-inflicted interruptions to occur. The risk of idle fingers touching controls they should not touch, in addition to individuals placing themselves in a compromised safety position, all points to a failure to appreciate the part everyone plays in maintaining a reduced risk environment.

Closure or interruption   8.11

Other examples of service interruption that might require the invocation of a coordinated response through the service continuity plan may include temporary closure of a maternity unit, or the accident and emergency unit or perhaps simultaneous failure of a number of life support systems. The duration of closure or interruption is one of the factors to consider when considering the impact and therefore the appropriateness of any contingency arrangement.

Incident creep   8.12

Without embarking on a prescriptive policy, it is useful for staff to have an aide-memoir setting out in broad terms what may be considered as a minor incident in order to differentiate it from a major incident. It is also important to get across the fact that incident creep can be a real issue – a minor incident without adequate response and control can become a major incident which eventually becomes much more difficult to control. So while demarcation between levels of incident can be useful, the cardinal rule with incident management, regardless of scale, is to attempt to gain control as soon as possible. Better to put in place a team to manage early, only to find that the situation can be addressed by line management, than to have senior management wishing they had put a team together hours previously.

Ideally, central coordination of what might be termed 'issues management' needs to be established. Locally, a manager may be unaware that while they are dealing with a major issue, others in the organisation may be dealing with similar or equally serious matters. Could it be that if the incidents are considered together, the service continuity plan should be put on standby or brought into play? Someone needs to be aware of all incidents and to manage service continuity from this holistic angle. It is best to encourage management to have local contingency arrangements for their service units, but when failure of the entire service unit is likely as a result of the incident, the service continuity plan should be invoked.

The impact of service interruption   8.13

Essentially, the impact of interruption on service delivery must be measured in terms of two components:

- scale; and
- duration.

In other words, every organisation has a tolerance level beyond which pain is experienced. In the health sector the pain is usually expressed in service down-time, patient complaint or poor outcome for the patient.

The scale of the interruption will range from affecting only one unit through to widespread disruption, and will depend on the delay before service can be resumed. The time period can have an impact in scale from inconvenient to life threatening.

Loss of facilities 8.14

Take the example of a complete failure of the centralised steam boiler. What impact will this have on a hospital's ability to function?

The absence of heating and hot water will be immediately critical for patients and staff and alternative arrangements will have to be made quickly. However, for some services – such as outpatients – it may be sufficient to arrange a local radio announcement indicating the intention to resume normal services in a few days' time.

Alternatively, consider control rooms and their communication facilities – can these be replicated off-site, or diverted to alternative facilities? Are there centralised environmental controls for heat, light, and water supplies? Should there be a sanctioned alternative arrangement?

What if an incident extends beyond 24 hours? Take fire or an asbestos contaminated building – will there be an exponential increase in the services affected?

Loss of staff 8.15

The questions posed above concern the physical environment, but the healthcare sector has no greater asset than its people. Contingency plans must consider the impact of loss of staff. Annual influenza out-breaks affect not just the public but also staff. A major accident involving large number of individuals and serious loss of life has very traumatic consequences and requires a unique sensitivity. Organisations should ensure that service continuity plans include plans to cope with reduced staffing levels, and post-incident management and communication.

Resources 8.16

The larger the concern over the business impact, the greater the resources needed to cope with the consequences. Resources are not only financial – more often than not, it is about having the right people in the right place at the right time. The speed of attendance may be a key factor but so also is competency – and it all comes back to preparedness. A suitable level of preparedness involves training in substitute equipment and methods of working. Clearly not all potential incidents present a common impact and therefore the level of resources and urgency of response for each will vary.

Getting the balance right is difficult, but it is a decision that must be made, periodically reviewed and adjusted by senior management. Often it is a judgment call because not all major incidents clearly manifest their implications immediately. A fire or major building failure may be the exception.

With careful thought, it is not difficult to imagine the impact of a major incident, yet it is not something that many in senior management seem to consider without being prompted during a service continuity management project.

Business impact: strategic principles 8.17

Why not consider what a disaster would mean, in the cool light of day? A number of strategic principles need to be considered:

- Can the organisation prioritise its response to an incident?
- Are some services more critical than others?
- Which services would the organisation defend at all costs?
- What are the factors influencing such a selection of priorities?
- What are the political, reputational, geographical, financial and demographic influences?
- Who might need to know about an incident?
- What would the organisation say in defence of its actions?
- What might be the consequences of such a statement?
- Who else will be involved?
- Who would the organisation want to involve?
- Who does the organisation want to make sure is not involved?

This thought process can form the basis for considering a management strategy. This strategy needs to be clear about its aims. If the aim is known it is much easier to focus on achieving an agreed course of management actions or objectives.

The next step is to convey the strategy to staff at all levels. They need to make a commitment to mitigation activity from identified threats, agree the appropriate level of preparedness and have confidence in organisation-wide and departmental service continuity plans to reduce the impact of an interruption.

Developing service continuity plans 8.18

Under the direction of hospital accident and emergency units, major incident plans have been in place for many years, to cope professionally and sensitively with disasters. These plans sit alongside local authorities' generic emergency plans involving the emergency services, social services and other statutory and voluntary organisations.

Such plans are intended to cope, for example, with a weather event, a community calamity, an explosion or a transport accident. Depending upon the degree of involvement and professional expertise required, some plans require more detail than others. In the same way, healthcare providers need to develop a range of internal action plans to ensure continuity of service.

Internal action plans   8.19

Internal action plans are based on the premise that continuity of service provision to the local community is a prerequisite, not least because:

- the population's tolerance of service interruption is ever-diminishing;

- maintenance of the trust or service provider's reputation, in the eyes of the public and the health authority, is essential; and

- the chief executive has to satisfy elected representatives and trust board members that in the event of an emergency all is being done that can be done.

Three phases of response   8.20

A clearly thought out and predetermined action plan involving all staff at all levels needs to be implemented, including the strategic response of senior management in a crisis management plan, as well as a detailed functional or tactical response of departmental staff in their service recovery plan. By breaking the evolution of the incident down into three defined phases (see **FIGURE 8.1**) it is possible to allocate responsibilities and inform staff where they fit in.

Figure 8.1: Three phases of response

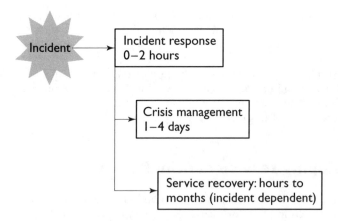

The people involved 8.21

Before embarking on a service continuity project it is essential to ensure the project has the sponsorship of the chief executive, or most senior manager, and that the project is not seen as yet another initiative over which heads of directorates and departments can prioritise their attention. In today's working environment there is real danger in project overload. It is therefore essential that the project is monitored at the highest level and those involved are supported.

When developing functional service continuity plans it is important to have directorate and department heads on board throughout, and to this end, it is prudent to have a project steering group. This should include the senior management team, since they already have a firm grasp of the organisation's strategic direction and its key responsibilities in an external incident. It can be useful to demonstrate that external major accident plans can be used as a basis, subject to modification, for the creation of internal service continuity plans.

Keep it simple 8.22

For a plan to work, it must be simple and easy to use. A complete version will be held by the plan coordinator and team leaders, but individual members of the teams, with specific responsibilities, need only have, for example, their actions recorded on a laminated A4 card.

It must be remembered that the plan will be used in a stressful situation by individuals, each of whom will bring to the event their own frame of mind and level of competence. This should be borne in mind when selecting the language and phraseology used in the plan. It must reflect the culture and terminology of the organisation and not introduce a new vocabulary.

Life cycle 8.23

Typically service continuity management should establish and then repeat a life cycle of phased activities. First, the steering group must decide where in the life cycle it considers the organisation to be in the development of its service continuity management culture. The lifecycle can be portrayed as in FIGURE 8.2.

Figure 8.2: The service continuity management life cycle

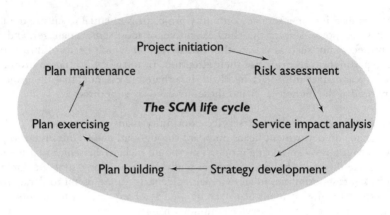

Project initiation 8.24

This first stage of a service continuity programme involves obtaining commitment from senior management and project personnel to agree the scope, objectives, method, timing, work schedule and budget. It also involves examination of the existing tolerance to interruption in different aspects of the organisation, and produces an incident definition and high-level incident management command and control structure.

Risk assessment 8.25

Organisations adopting the NHS controls assurance standards (SEE 8.52) will be familiar with the development of a risk register. Integral to the process must be an element of risk assessment. This is the basis on which all of the organisation's risks are identified, evaluated and given a score or ranking in terms of impact and likelihood. The exercise facilitates a mechanism to manage risk in the organisation across a whole range of issues, typically grouped into three risk categories:

- **Strategic risk** – reputation, service offering, political direction.

- **Operational risk** – personnel, health and safety, property assets, healthcare procedures.

- **Financial risk** – budget controls, contract terms.

At the end of the exercise a report outlining the identified risk areas can be presented to the board which will enable them to make informed loss mitigation choices.

Frequently, where a formal risk assessment and register has not been commissioned, organisations will cherry-pick their risks for attention, based on whatever is apparently most pressing. This is not ideal because underlying root causes are not addressed. The board really ought to expend its resources in a professional and transparent way consistent with corporate governance and controls assurance. To do this a full register of risks is required.

The risk assessment process is a useful prelude to the service continuity process because it can point to the major risks that should be considered in the impact analysis stage. There is one proviso, however: when considering interruption to services the concept of probability or likelihood is unhelpful. A risk may be classified as a one in a 100-year event, but what if it occurred tomorrow?

A risk register should be used for base information, but the impact of loss should be reconsidered in the service impact analysis (SIA) stage. It is about considering the big catastrophic risks to the organisation – not just physical risks.

Service impact analysis 8.26

The SIA considers the critical processes in an organisation and assesses the impact of the risks identified in the risk assessment. Essentially it is about listing all that is done under normal conditions.

Each process is considered in relation to all other functions, and then prioritised in order of recovery to minimise the damage to service continuity in the event of an incident. In addition, upstream and downstream interdependencies, mitigation or protection arrangements, and the current state of preparedness, if any, for recovery are examined.

Recovery options must be considered, minimum post-loss resource requirements identified, and recovery milestones along a timeline introduced.

Recovery strategy 8.27

Agreeing a service continuity strategy is only the first step. For successful implementation, financial and staff resources will be necessary. Certain items might need to be purchased, installed and linked to existing processes. Contracts might need to be entered into with third parties, or other arrangements put in place, such as mutual aid or reciprocal agreements.

Staff will probably require training, given that for some the handling of an emergency situation will be alien to their usual day job. Certainly, work around methods for current practice will need to be agreed – such as alternative procedures to resuscitate a hospital patient should the defibrillators malfunction simultaneously.

The formation of a service continuity strategy demonstrates the security of the organisation's critical processes to stakeholders. It also gives the senior management group an opportunity to benchmark their recovery strategies against healthcare standards.

Plan writing   8.28

The plan will be used by ordinary people at all organisational levels and must, therefore, be easily comprehensible. One moment they may be operating in normal conditions, the next potentially in chaos. The plan should be snappy and easy to use. In the first instance, the concern is to learn the facts – the what, why, where, when, and who. Those called upon to react can often be faced with sensory overload. Why not establish responsibilities and communication channels in advance and determine who needs to know and when?

Five requirements of a sound plan   8.29

On the basis of a sound command and control structure, a plan can be condensed into five main sections:

- corporate policy and incident command and control;

- emergency response in the first hours following an incident;

- crisis management in the first days following an incident;

- service recovery from day one until the full recovery of the organisation; and

- contact details listing who needs to be told and where assistance is to be sought.

Corporate policy and incident command and control   8.30

The introduction to the plan must contain minimal detail. Users of a plan should be familiar with the history of the plan's development; while the plan coordinator will have good reason to detail a background and plan maintenance records, these are not required in an incident and can be placed in an alternative document. What is needed here is a quick reminder of how the plan will work and who will be responsible for what action.

Emergency response in the first hours following an incident   8.31

This element of the plan is location-specific and forms a tactical response to an immediate situation. It could be a physical event such as loss of power or accommodation, but equally it could be an IT failure, or perhaps a serious complaint with the potential for impact on an organisation's reputation. The team involved in emergency response should be drawn from across the organisation and may co-opt assistance beyond the team as the occasion dictates.

Crisis management in the first days following an incident   8.32

This is the strategic response to a report of an incident coming from the emergency response team, which should comprise members of the senior management team. Their objective must be to be able to pull back from the immediate response activity and consider strategic issues and implications. Essentially they must consider where does this situation place the organisation in terms of its operational objectives, responsibilities and its vision statement? In the light of this requirement the team needs to establish a command centre as the hub of management activity.

The most critical aspect of their work is communication to all the stakeholders in the community and in the organisation itself. It is from the command centre that press and media response should be coordinated. The strategic direction and the pre-agreed recovery strategies will require regular review and, potentially, modification in light of the situation as it evolves. Ultimately return to a position of some normality within a week is needed even if it means working from temporary accommodation.

Interestingly, the impact of a disaster or major incident can be the first occasion when the calibre of the management team is actually observed by an external constituency. It is therefore essential for the preservation of the organisation and its directors to be seen to be able to handle such an event competently. Media training is a prerequisite.

Service recovery from day one until the full recovery of the organisation   8.33

This element of the service continuity plan is crucial. Using a generic template, filling in the boxes without understanding the need, is a recipe for failure. Building upon the foundation work done in the service impact analysis, alternative arrangements to deliver continuity of service can be recorded for each of the organisation's functions.

Clearly where a major interruption has occurred, access may be denied to accommodation or staff are unable to fulfil their roles, it will be impossible to restore all functions simultaneously. That is why it is important to rank the order of recovery in terms of priority. In addition, an understanding of knock-on effects can be gleaned from an interdependency study.

At the end of the exercise each directorate or department should have their own version of the plan, specific to their area. A composite plan will be held at the command centre and by the plan coordinator.

Contact details listing who needs to be told and where assistance is to be sought 8.34

A comprehensive database of contacts must be developed. Not surprisingly, this is the one element of the plan, which is constantly changing and should be regularly reviewed.

Plans often focus on the specific recovery of critical service provision. Each section of the plan must consider who is involved, their roles, responsibilities and what action is likely to be needed, how this is to be carried out and in what order. The plan needs to be flexible and action-oriented. Planning for the worst eventuality – typically a denied access situation – means the plan will meet the needs of any situation.

Plan exercising 8.35

To write a plan is only the first step. Few plans in their first appearance are fully satisfactory.

It is essential to prove to the teams that what has been written will meet the objectives of recovery and service continuity. The use of the term 'exercising' is deliberate. It is not about testing or giving marks out of ten. It is about rehearsing the people through their action steps and giving them experience of working in an out-of-the-ordinary situation and one which is potentially very stressful.

Plan exercising can range from a talk through to full simulation, including evacuation of the site, full exercise of the plan and media exposure of senior management.

Component-level exercising 8.36

Exercising should be done in component level to start with; it is never wise to try and do a full simulation of the whole plan as a first event. It is necessary to build up competence levels in all the teams and sort out the apparent difficulties of each before bringing them together.

One component, which is easy to do, and will reveal any communication weaknesses in the plan, is to exercise the call cascade or contact list in the plan. On the basis of those individuals able to respond to a phone call over a weekend, for example, it can be determine how easily the plan can be implemented. Many plans fail at the first hurdle because the phone number is not correct or there is no out-of-hours contact number. The retention of individual phone numbers and email addresses are a useful addition to the contact armoury.

Plan exercising identifies the improvement areas required in the plan, and provides hands-on experience for all staff involved. It validates the work done to date and, if done correctly, will ensure that no team or group of individuals is more advanced in their state of preparedness than others.

Plan maintenance   8.37

The maintenance of the service continuity plan is as crucial as its development. Nobody writes an operating performance plan for one financial year to have it gather dust in the next. It is constantly reviewed and updated in the light of the operating environment. The same must apply to a service continuity plan. Ideally managers should see its maintenance as part of their responsibilities consistent with the controls assurance programme and corporate governance requirements.

If exercising is done on a regular basis (at least annually) then it can be expected that the plan will automatically require updating and refining. Certainly managers should be encouraged to review their plan biannually looking, in particular, to ensure the document reflects the current service offering, since in some instances this may have changed since the plan was first written.

Implementation of service continuity plans   8.38

The vision at all times is of a plan that is easily usable by all levels in an organisation, even under adverse conditions. Staff will not want to use large lever-arch file plans, which are heavy in descriptive text, under such circumstances.

As previously discussed, the plans can be structured under the headings of:

* emergency response,
* crisis management; and
* service recovery.

This gives the senior management team a clear picture.

Development of a service continuity plan is initially resource-hungry, until such time as it can be signed off, subject to modification through rehearsal and exercising. Like any project that is worth doing, management and staff should be clear on the deliverables and timescale to achieve them.

Sometimes there can be objections to putting these resources together. In addition, there may be cost implications. The use of external resources to assist the project, lend it weight and deliver a tried and tested methodology can be seen as a cost. A more positive perspective will be to see it as an investment.

External assistance   8.39

External assistance can be very useful and usually comes in two forms: consultancy and software.

Consultancy   8.40

Engaging a consultant should be done after examining their credentials. A track record in service continuity should be expected, and previous experience in the healthcare sector would be useful. It is worth enquiring as to their adherence to the 10 standards advocated by the Business Continuity Institute as listed below:

Ten standards of the Business Continuity Institute:

1.   Project initiation and management.

2.   Risk evaluation and control.

3.   Business impact analysis.

4.   Developing business continuity strategies.

5.   Emergency response and operations.

6.   Developing and implementing business continuity plans.

7.   Awareness and training programmes.

8.   Maintaining and exercising business continuity plans.

9.   Public relations and crisis coordination.

10.   Coordination with public authorities.

Their competency must be ascertained. Do they come with a technical or information systems bias or a wider organisational focus? Remember the subtle distinction between disaster recovery of the IT system as distinct from service continuity management of the whole organisation.

There is no doubt that a consultant will bring to the organisation a range of tried and tested methodologies and personal experience drawn from many industries and sectors, which, with careful agreement with the organisation's plan coordinator, should minimise the amount of management input required, whilst maintaining sufficient ownership. Some consultancies will encourage the use of bespoke planning software while others prefer using the office packages in common use. There is no hard and fast rule.

Software   8.41

Software can be useful, particularly where an internal plan coordinator has limited experience and is quite keen on an IT solution. There are, however, some drawbacks. What you get is what you see. These are off-the-shelf packages and customisation will be down to the user. It will be up to the user to use whatever parts of the software they deem appropriate. If they are not entirely sure what they want to achieve, there is a danger that a fill-in-the-box approach may be adopted without due care, resulting in critical parts of a plan being omitted or undue attention to material that is not essential.

Complex inter-relationship databases can be very clever, but it does rather lock the plan coordinator into being the author, editor and reviser for all future versions of the plan. This could be quite a workload and reduces the opportunity for sharing ownership of the planning process. The plan ought to be owned by all managers and recognised by their staff.

Ideally, the plan coordinator wants to engage the whole organisation and therefore present the plan in a format that is familiar to the end user. This leads to a coordination management role enabling a more holistic approach to training, exercising, maintenance and auditing programmes.

Rebutting objections   8.42

Regardless of the approach adopted, there are bound to be objections from some quarters. It might therefore be helpful to present some of the arguments here and suggest some rebuttals.

We can't afford it we don't need it   8.43

Can your organisation afford to be without a service continuity plan? Can directors ignore their corporate governance responsibilities? Research has shown that effective continuity management greatly reduces post-disaster losses. It also brings additional advantage in encouraging a broader risk management culture.

It requires too much management time   8.44

Management involvement is essential to ensure proper ownership of the project and delivery to schedule. Ideally, the project coordinator should look to spread the load across the organisation.

We've done disaster recovery   8.45

Service continuity management is more than disaster recovery. Disaster recovery is focused upon IT, whereas service continuity management looks across the whole of the organisation.

We already have a plan   8.46

Has it been exercised or audited? Would it stand up to a benchmark review? Can you be sure the format is suitable for use in a crisis? If you have any doubts about your existing plan, now is the time to engage a review before it is found wanting in a real and stressful situation.

Putting service continuity plans into practice   8.47

It is often stated that a plan must be a living document. The core ingredient of any workable plan is a robust and comprehensive command, control and communication protocol. Plans should be action-oriented, yet strategic, looking across the whole of the organisation, while usable at working level within individual departments. They should be focused upon loss of key functional ability from whatever cause, rather than being related to specific incidents. Ideally, the team which builds the plan will be the team called upon to implement it in the event of a real incident.

So where does the theory meet with the practice? A plan lying on the shelf in a director's office is no use – it just gathers dust. What is required is a programme of training and rehearsal that reduces the unknown element and surprise often experienced by those with little or no previous experience. One team gaining experience at the expense of others in the organisation is also counter-productive.

Plan components   8.48

As demonstrated in this chapter, the service continuity plan is actually a group of plans. Each can be seen as a component of the whole. Circumstances may dictate that it is appropriate in certain instances to use one component at a time, for example, to bring the crisis management team together for a significant event, however generally they are interrelated.

It is important to recognise the component nature of the plan in relation to the principal teams, that is:

- emergency response;
- crisis management; and
- departmental recovery.

Training   8.49

The next step is to train each team in its role and clearly amplify their responsibilities as detailed in the plan.

FIGURE 8.3 shows the effectiveness of a service continuity training programme that will raise the levels of competence equally across the organisation. While it could be argued that some training is better than none, the left chart is not as effective as the right.

Figure 8.3: Levels of training in different teams

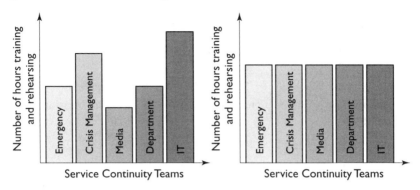

Effective training needs to be imaginative but realistic. There is little point in the UK of running a scenario involving an earthquake or tornado. People like to have a reference point, so a realistic scenario perhaps involving the breakdown of the central laundry, kitchen or energy centre is a good starting point.

Preparedness   8.50

Who will be the first to recognise an incident? What should be their reaction? Does the plan detail who should be informed and when? What will the informed person's reaction be?

In the emergency team it is a good idea to revolve the first on the call-out list. This enables more than a few to experience the leadership required in the plan. That way holidays, illness and attendance at conferences can be covered. Essentially the revolving role of leader in both the emergency and crisis team can be equated to the passing of the baton in a relay race.

By developing the scenario other facets of the plan will be highlighted. Who in the organisation is good at media handling? Is further training needed from specialists in this area? Will the timeline on the recovery of the IT systems and applications marry with the end user requirements and their recovery timeline?

By encouraging a culture of training and preparedness within the organisation, there is no doubt the teams will be able to handle the unexpected competently and robustly. Not only that, they will have tangible proof of their compliance with the controls assurance programme which can in turn be demonstrated to their stakeholders.

A strategic investment 8.51

Any successful modern organisation strives to achieve optimum service through a combination of the right strategy and maximisation of its resources. We have seen this in the healthcare sector in a number of ways:

- corporate restructuring – creation, merging and de-merging of trusts;

- strategies to address increased utilisation of staff and mission-critical resources;

- commercial integration or partnership with third-party suppliers;

- implementation of just-in-time processes;

- a focus on quality as well as value;

- compliance with governance programmes, sector regulations and requirements;

- changes in strategic direction or the introduction of new services;

- complex interdependencies and a growing reliance on third parties in the delivery of service; and

- increased communication with more demanding stakeholders.

Critical to the success of many of these initiatives is good project management, and integral to the project management approach must be a recognition of the part played by corporate governance and risk management in general and service continuity in particular. Service continuity management is a vital component in the delivery of these strategies, as well as a key discipline in the successful day-to-day management of any organisation. Service continuity strategies must link directly with what matters in delivering a level of service to the public.

For an organisation valuing its people, running critical IT and facilities, and investing in its reputation and community perception, service continuity represents a comparatively small investment in exchange for operational security and peace of mind.

In an increasingly intolerant world, a successful service continuity programme is often a source of distinct reputational advantage. The alternative is an unprepared organisation displaying its inefficiencies in an unsuccessfully managed interruption for all the world to watch.

Service continuity management as part of the holistic risk management programme must be seen as a strategic investment, not a cost, involving all layers within the organisation.

NHS Executive controls assurance standards – non-clinical 8.52

1. Risk management system

2. Buildings, land plant, and non-medical equipment

3. Catering and food hygiene

4. Contracts and control of contractors

5. Emergency preparedness

6. Environmental management

7. Fire safety

8. Health and safety management

9. Human resources

10. Infection control

11. Information management and technology

12. Medical devices management

13. Medicines management

14. Professional and product liability

15. Records management

16. Security

17. Transport

18. Waste management

19. De-contamination

Useful websites

Business Continuity Institute: *www.thebci.com*

Government Emergency Planning Division: *www.homeoffice.gov.uk/epd*

Offrisk Consulting Ltd: www.offrisk.com

Online services

Crisis navigator (internet guide to crisis management): *www.crisisnavigator.org*

www.disasterplan.com

Emergencynet (online emergency news and analysis): *www.emergency.com*

Globalcontinuity.com (information on business risk and continuity planning): *www.globalcontinuity.com*

Courses and literature

Glasgow Caledonian University: *www.gcal.ac.uk*

Rothstein Associates Inc (book and software catalogue): *www.rothstein.com*

Scarman Centre at the University of Leicester: *www.le.ac.uk/scarman/cp.html*

University of Sheffield: *www.shef.ac.uk*

Chapter 9
Managing People

This chapter covers:

- Workforce expansion.

- Lessons from high-profile reports.

- Recruitment and selection procedures.

- Induction training, appraisal and revalidation.

- Leadership and management training.

- Staff retention and morale.

- The statutory framework.

Introduction   9.1

CHAPTER 2 defines risk management and the strategies for managing risk as part of organisational processes. It shows that risk management is a learning process and how organisations must understand the causes of risk in order to then introduce proper control measures. The links with quality and high standards of care provision are also explored.

Managing change   9.2

The organisation of healthcare in the UK is subject to constant change. Whenever change is planned, the human resource management priority is to identify the issues, by which we generally mean the constraints, problems and the risks. The risks are those arising from not getting it right, both in terms of statutory requirements (for example, consultation and employee transfers), but also in managing the people affected so that effective and safe delivery of services continue.

People management processes   9.3

Similarly, from the point of view of the daily running of health services, there are issues, or risks, arising from people management processes. Processes affecting an employee's journey through an organisation, from recruitment and induction, through appraisal and development, to termination arrangements, can lead to risks if not carried out effectively.

This chapter aims to explore this journey, and to examine how risks can arise at different stages, the potential impact on employee behaviour and on the organisation and successful healthcare delivery. It also aims to address the human resource solutions to these risks, and to offer practical advice to managers in handling the situations and risks which can arise when managing people.

The link between staff and service   9.4

Risk management spans all functions in organisations. Effective people management underpins the reduction of risk in healthcare and links into clinical governance and improving the quality of care for patients. Recent research from Aston University[1] has found a strong connection between Human Resource (HR) management, and lower patient mortality. This particularly applies in organisations where staff work in teams, there are training policies in place for all staff and sophisticated appraisal schemes. The practical aspects of these key elements are explored further in this chapter.

One of the core principles embodied in the NHS Plan (see **KEY REFERENCES, APPENDIX 1**) is the need to work continuously to improve health services and to minimise errors. The link between high-quality staff, quality services and reducing errors is a major theme of current thinking, carried forward into the national goal for every healthcare organisation to be a model employer through good human resource management.

Workforce expansion

Investment in staff   9.5

The NHS Plan announced expansion in staff numbers by 2004, comprising 20,000 more nurses, 7,500 more consultants, 2,000 more GPs and 6,500 more therapists and other health professionals, to meet its overall goals for achieving improvements in the quality of healthcare. National human resource strategies[2] recognise that recruitment is not the only solution to achieving workforce expansion. There needs to be investment in staff in order to produce a quality workforce. This means modernising professional education and training, and introducing family-friendly employment policies to ensure that scarce healthcare skills and expertise are not lost.

Restoring public confidence   9.6

Underlying this is also the need to restore public confidence in the delivery of healthcare. High-profile reports on events at Bristol Royal Infirmary (see **KEY**

REFERENCES, APPENDIX 1) and the Royal Liverpool Children's Hospital identi-fied key failings, including in people management. Similarly, the Clothier Report (SEE **9.8**)and Bullock Report (SEE **9.11**)(analysed below) into the issues arising from the activities of individual health workers, and other reports concerning GP and locum appointments, highlighted risks in traditional practice. Although these reports relate to clinical staff, the problems identified, and the action to raise stan-dards are equally applicable to other healthcare workers.

There are human resource management solutions to many of the risks identified in the reports, including recommendations on recruitment, selection, training, appraisal, supervision and leadership. It is important to learn from these experi-ences, and incorporate their lessons into strategies for good employment practice for all healthcare workers, in order to manage the risks arising from individual behaviour or organisational failings.

Lessons from Allitt and others   9.7

Over the last ten years or so there have been a number of incidents where the actions of individuals have resulted in patient harm and public concern about the safety of care. These all have lessons for human resource practitioners in the same way as they have for other healthcare managers and professionals.

The report of the inquiry into the case of enrolled nurse Beverley Allitt[3] describes how during early 1991 there was a series of incidents on the children's ward at Grantham Hospital. Three children died suddenly on the ward and one at home not long after discharge. Nine other children collapsed unexpectedly, some more than once.

In many of the cases it seemed to the ward doctors that what had happened was unusual, but could be explained on the basis of the children's medical history. Nevertheless, suspicion grew that these might be cases of deliberate harm. A police investigation took place, and Beverley Allitt was charged with four mur-ders and nine attempted murders.

The Clothier report   9.8

The Clothier report into the case was critical of both senior management in the hospital, and nurse management on the ward for failing to act when suspicions first arose.

Criticisms   9.9

The report also found the background to the employment of Beverley Allitt as an enrolled nurse was 'unsatisfactory'. She had an exceptionally high level of sickness absence as a student nurse, missing 126 days during the nurse-training course, and was later found to display evidence of a major personality disorder. Yet her health record was disregarded, and referral for assessment by the occupational health department was neglected.

The managerial procedures for the appointment itself were described as 'sloppy'. There were no records of an application form being completed, and no written references. The personnel department was not informed of her appointment, and there were delays in issuing a contract of employment. Beverley Allitt had started work before any health screening took place, and despite the requirement for managers to check that a candidate has no previous criminal convictions before appointment to a post with substantial access to children, no police check was made. In fact she had no previous convictions, but the inquiry found the failure to follow normal procedures 'extremely worrying'.

Recommendations   9.10

The recommendations of the inquiry included the following on nurse appointments:

- In addition to routine references, the most recent employer or place of study should be asked to provide at least a record of time taken off on grounds of sickness.

- No candidate for nursing in whom there is evidence of major personality disorder should be employed in the profession.

- Nurses should undergo formal health screening when they obtain their first posts after qualifying.

The case of Beverley Allitt is an extreme one, and the report acknowledges:

'No measures can afford complete protection against a determined miscreant. The main lesson from the inquiry, and our principle recommendation, is that the Grantham disaster should serve to heighten awareness in all those caring for children of the possibility of malevolent intervention as a cause of unexpected critical events.'

The case is a good example of how low risk probability can have a high impact in terms of consequences to patient care and damage to public confidence. This is also seen in the following reports.

The Bullock report   9.11

This report[4] looked at the case of Amanda Jenkinson, who was employed as a nurse in the intensive therapy unit at Bassetlaw District General Hospital, and in January 1994 was alleged to have tampered with equipment on the unit, putting patients at risk. She was suspended from duty and a series of investigations took place extending over several years. These resulted in a police prosecution, a conviction for serious assault and a prison sentence.

Failure to report medical history 9.12

Amanda Jenkinson was dismissed by the trust in 1995, not for any action while on the intensive therapy unit, but for an alleged failure to report fully her medical history. The report of the independent inquiry set up by North Nottinghamshire Health Authority states:

> 'A determined and devious deceiver will always be difficult to detect, but a series of nets to catch such an employee or recruit could be constructed by means of cross-checking information from the applicant against that given by previous employers, occupational health departments and the employee's GP.'

The report notes that although the hospital obtained references from previous employers, they were let down by the nature of the references which, seen retrospectively, were ambiguous and did not deal with the problems encountered by these previous employers. Taking references supplied to other trusts together, the report says, a pattern emerges of a character with difficulty accepting guidance, discipline or superior authority.

Recommendations 9.13

A number of recommendations are made on references, including that a standard form should be used, and that references should deal with fact rather than impressions. Where impressions are conveyed, factual examples or evidence should substantiate those impressions.

The report also recommends greater consistency in interview techniques and documentation, and the training of all those involved in the recruitment and selection process. A structured process with probing, relevant questions at interview would almost certainly have picked up the earlier concerns, and enabled them to be tested and verified.

General practice 9.14

Harold Shipman, a Manchester GP, was convicted in January 2000 of the murders of 15 elderly women in his care. A Department of Health audit of his career later found that he recorded 297 more deaths of patients than other doctors, 236 of which were at home. An Independent Public Inquiry is taking place to establish what changes to current systems are needed in order to safeguard patients in the future. The Inquiry's first reports have been published with recommendations on whistleblowing, disciplinary systems and selection procedures.

The Commission for Health Improvement (CHI) inquiry report (SEE **CHI WEBSITE**) into the case of Peter Green, a Loughborough GP found guilty of abusing patients, says there must be a more open and honest system for appointing GPs. The introduction of standard systems for the appointment of GPs, whether as partners or single-handed practitioners, is more difficult because of their independent employment status. However, all appointments should follow the good practice processes outlined in this chapter, with proper checks made. Outside assessors should be involved to ensure independent, professional scrutiny and avoid the risk these cases highlight.

Employing locum consultants

The Elwood case   9.15

James Elwood was a retired consultant who worked as a short-term locum in several NHS hospitals. Concerns arose about discrepancies between his histopathology reports and the findings of other clinicians, but not before a number of patients had received inappropriate treatment as a result of errors in diagnosis, with serious consequences in seven cases.

The Secretary of State for Health asked CHI to investigate the use of locum medical practitioners in four NHS trusts, with particular reference to Dr Elwood. The report[5] notes that the case has been the subject of considerable national and local publicity. It generated public and professional concern about medical errors and locum doctors. It also raises several important issues for the health service about the recruitment and management of doctors who move around the service, working for short periods in different places, and how concerns about clinical competence are communicated between employers.

Like others in England and Wales, the four trusts investigated by CHI make use of locum medical practitioners at various levels of seniority to cover holiday and study leave, unfilled posts, and to supplement staff at times of particular pressure. Appointments are usually needed at very short notice and for a relatively short time (days or weeks). There is a temptation not to be as thorough as for permanent appointments, but the risks, as the Elwood case shows, are just as great.

CHI report   9.16

The CHI report found that reliance on locum consultants is frequently due to poor workforce planning, particularly in terms of arrangements for covering leave for permanent consultants, and is often a substitute for the appointment of additional permanent consultants. In the field of histopathology, such problems are compounded by a shortage of qualified consultants.

Appointment   9.17

There is a NHS Code of Practice[6] on the appointment of locum doctors, but CHI found the four trusts concerned consistently failed to comply with these requirements, and meet their duty of care to patients in employing doctors of proven ability to fulfil their responsibilities. The report describes how the trusts failed to use adequate safeguards when obtaining references, checking career history, interviewing, carrying out health checks and during induction.

Performance monitoring   9.18

Performance monitoring of locum consultants was also found to be poor, with little systematic checking of the quality or accuracy of their work. CHI recommends that locums should be subject to the same system of clinical audit and performance monitoring as their permanent colleagues. There should be routine checking of locum consultants' work by an identified clinical supervisor and early notification of the medical director when errors or a pattern of poor practice are identified.

Communication between trusts   9.19

CHI also found a serious problem in ensuring that concerns about the performance or conduct of locum doctors are communicated between trusts and around the NHS generally. Too often the solution is to terminate employment, without advising other healthcare employers that there may be a risk. This is likely to be covered by new arrangements.

The Bristol inquiry (Kennedy report)   9.20

The risk outcome from an episode such as that at Bristol Royal Infirmary (see KEY REFERENCES, APPENDIX 1) is the consequential damage to the organisation's reputation and the professionals involved. The patient safety issues also have lessons for human resource practitioners.

The case   9.21

This was the largest ever investigation into clinical practice in the NHS, triggered by infant deaths during surgery in the late 1980s and early 1990s. Despite concerns about death rates raised by a whistleblower, by colleagues and by parents, surgeons at the Bristol Royal Infirmary failed to recognise or admit this, and continued to operate.

Culture   9.22

How did this happen? Culture has already been identified as a high-risk area for any organisation, and the inquiry report found too much arrogance, ambition and muddling through at the hospital, with a 'club culture' which shut out young doctors. A blame culture in particular contributed to senior doctors' refusal to recognise that mistakes were being made. The Health Secretary said: 'If the NHS is to learn when things go wrong, it must move beyond a culture of blame.' Introduction of audit and appraisal, (SEE **9.66**), are key outcomes.

227

Skills   9.23

The report also cites the lack of requirement for consultants to keep their skills up to date. 'Once qualified, the prevailing view was that it was up to them to maintain their competence save in exceptional circumstances... . The hospital consultant effectively has a job for life.'

Accountability   9.24

Accountability is a key issue in understanding the nature of risk. The relationship between clinicians and managers often focuses on volume of clinical activity, with too little concept of accountability to an employer; rather the concept of clinical freedom assumes doctors are accountable to their patients to obtain the best for them. Yet it is a reasonable assumption that the board of a trust should take steps to assess the risk to the public, and is responsible if the public is not adequately protected.

Further points   9.25

There are two other important points from the inquiry on the people agenda:

- The NHS must put patients at its core. They must be treated with respect – this requires a cultural, behavioural and attitude change.

- Care must be as safe as possible – requiring good recruitment and selection, appraisal and training, revalidation and continuing professional development.

The DoH response in January 2002[7] summarises the action to be taken in detail.

The inquiry report also highlighted issues about teamworking and leadership. Poor teamwork had 'implications for performance and outcome'. The report says the relationship between the various professional groups was sometimes poor, demonstrating a lack of leadership. The medical director was described as having 'power but no leadership'.

Understaffing was also a factor, and this is developed further in the section on the need for adequate resources.

The Royal Liverpool inquiry   9.26

This inquiry[8] resulted from public concerns about the removal, retention, and disposal of human tissue and organs without proper consent or senior management knowledge of the extent of the practice. The report, published in January 2001, reiterates many issues about clinical governance covered in the Bristol inquiry. It also formulates management standards, three of which are relevant to people management, and are summarised in the recommendations as follows:

- No clinician should be appointed to a position of managerial authority in a hospital without having relevant clinical experience for the position.

- No clinician should take effective control of a management position until trained in all necessary management techniques and in any relevant legal requirements.

- Hospital managers should be of a suitable background and calibre for the role expected of them, provided with all the necessary training (including continued education) and themselves regularly appraised for the quality of their performance.

Major changes on consent are to be introduced; there will be training in organ retention and obtaining consent from relatives. Human resource managers have to ensure this training is incorporated into trust induction and other education programmes.

The Victoria Climbie Inquiry   9.27

This was the Inquiry into the child protection failings around the death of eight year old Victoria Climbie, who died following months of ill-treatment at home. The Inquiry was conducted by Lord Laming, who was particularly concerned about the low level of priority given to child protection by the agencies involved in the care of Victoria, and strongly criticised people in senior positions who denied their own responsibility.

The Commission for Health Improvement report[9] observes that skilled and competent frontline staff, adequate management support and professional supervision are crucial elements in child protection. In the case of the NHS organisations involved, there are comments about the timeliness and variable quality of care. Shortages of skilled and qualified staff in particular caused delays in allocating complex cases, and providing protected time for designated doctors and nurses to carry out their child protection roles could be a problem.

There was also an over reliance on agency staff, who were not properly checked through the Criminal Records Bureau, and did not receive adequate training.

Summary of the lessons learnt   9.28

The human resource lessons learnt from these inquiries and reports are summarised in the Table below. Many are recruitment issues, but others have a wider organisational context.

How these and other people management risk issues can be addressed, and used to enhance the value of people management to the business of the organisation, is examined in the remainder of the chapter.

Report/inquiry	Issues
Clothier report	Reference checking Occupational health involvement Interview technique Systems approach
Bullock report	Structured references Occupational health involvement Interview process Recruitment and selection training
General practice (CHI Report)	Appointment processes Checking qualifications and career history Whistle blowing Disciplinary procedures Fitness to practice checks
Use of locums	Recruitment processes Reference checks Career history checks Fitness to practise Alerting other employers Appraisal Identifying and learning from errors
Bristol Royal Infirmary (Kennedy report)	Culture Appraisal, revalidation and continuing professional development/skill updating Adequate resources Accountability Leadership
Royal Liverpool (Redfern Report)	Management appointment criteria Management training and continuing professional development Induction and staff training Culture
Victoria Climbie Inquiry (Laming Report)	Skill shortages Management support and capacity Training

Recruitment and selection procedures   9.29

Good recruitment and selection procedures are important for the proper protection of patients, other healthcare workers and the public as they ensure that people are qualified to do the job and have the right skills for today's complex healthcare world. The risks of making inappropriate appointments are seen in poor performance in the role, with increased risk of error, and in risks from failure to meet statutory obligations.

Recruitment is also expensive. The average cost of recruiting to a post in the public sector is nearly £4,000. The Chartered Institute of Personnel and Development estimates this cost can be over £6,000 per leaver in managerial positions. These costs include transition costs, for example unproductive time while learning or serving notice, and loss in customer service or 'satisfaction'. There is a further hidden cost, since on average, a new recruit only reaches their full potential when they have been in post for a year.[10]

So how can processes be enhanced, to address the lessons to be learnt from Allitt and others, to avoid unnecessary costs and to ensure trusts make safe appointments to all healthcare roles?

The purpose of recruitment is to attract applicants qualified for the jobs to be filled and the purpose of selection is to match applicants to those jobs. Most healthcare organisations have clear procedures for recruitment and selection, but it is worth summarising key good practice elements and commenting on some of the NHS and social policy trends that must also be taken into account.

Job description 9.30

Before any decision is made to advertise a job, the need and requirements of the role must be identified. Failure to do this adequately will result in inappropriate, costly appointments, leading to low productivity and high labour turnover. Developing a clear job description at this stage, in consultation with colleagues, sets out the role and its responsibilities, taking account of any changes required in the light of organisational design, costs, overlap of responsibilities and clinical risk. There must be constant review of job content and workload to make sure job descriptions are kept up to date and address responsibilities, including for managing risk areas.

Person specification 9.31

The person specification is derived from the job description and sets out the essential and desirable criteria required in the employee. In the NHS this increasingly takes a 'competency' approach. The term competency is used to describe work-related attributes such as the qualifications, skills, knowledge, experience and values that a person draws on in order to do their job well.

An accurate person specification is essential in order to attract people with the right qualifications, skills and experience. As we will see, the person specification is the basis for the rest of the procedure – if it is wrong, the rest of the procedure will also fail.

Attracting applicants 9.32

Employers must think about their strategy to reach the target recruitment market, and how to sell the job to people with the appropriate skills and qualifications. Most healthcare posts are advertised nationally in professional journals – it is a legal requirement for NHS consultant posts to be advertised in a minimum of two national journals – but there is increasing use of executive search and other external services.

In terms of the wider NHS strategy to increase workforce numbers, action nationally to improve recruitment processes includes:

• *Sharing strengths*, an NHS recruitment handbook published in June 2003, which promotes successful local campaigns and the national tools available.

• *Return to practice schemes* and evaluations to look at how many nurses completing return to work programmes come back and stay in the NHS.

• *NHS Careers website*, providing information for potential employees.

• *E-recruitment*, this service is being developed and will carry job advertisements and enable electronic application for jobs and training.

Equal opportunities 9.33

Employers also have to balance the need to match people to the person specification with national initiatives to encourage diversity. Employers who apply diversity policies recognise that a workforce that includes people from different social, cultural and educational backgrounds, age groups and the disabled can enrich the organisation and have a business impact. Inclusion policies enhance organisational performance in that poor targeting or indirect discrimination does not exclude good applicants.

Advertisements, job descriptions and person specifications must be free from any bias in terms of race, age and sex and other areas of discrimination, and from requirements unjustifiably excluding people with disabilities. All employers must have an equal opportunities policy to ensure statutory obligations are met (SEE **9.106** BELOW).

The recent NHS equal opportunities agreement, which aims to make equality and diversity part of everything the service does, requires open competition unless jobs are needed for redeployment – for example, to meet employer obligations regarding suitable alternative employment for employees at risk of redundancy, or if an employee becomes disabled. These policies, which meet legal obligations and ensure scarce skills are retained, have to be reconciled with clinical risk safeguards in placing people in new roles, achieved by training and good line management.

A national equalities and diversity strategy and delivery plan is being implemented to mainstream equality and diversity across the wider NHS, with one of its key aims to attract recruits from a wider cross section of the community.[11]

Selection process 9.34

The Office of the Commissioner for Public Appointments, identifies principles on which senior appointments must be based.[12] These are:

- merit;
- independent scrutiny;
- equal opportunities;
- probity;
- openness and transparency; and
- proportionality.

Applying these principles to healthcare appointments at all levels, in an appropriate way for the level of seniority and responsibility, will improve the quality of appointments and provide a strong defence to any later challenges. Processes must aim to deliver appointments on merit, meaning on the basis of how an individual's ability, experience and qualities match up to the person specification, with an appropriate degree of objective assessment.

In practical terms this means objective shortlisting processes to determine who will be selected for interview. Applicants should be matched to the person specification criteria by means of a scoring system, and the outcome recorded.

Effective interviews 9.35

The selection process itself must be designed to identify the candidates who are qualified to do the job. There has been much criticism of the interview as a selection tool, because of the risk of low objectivity. Research continues to find that employers recruit people they like rather than the people with the best skills for the job. Many still use 'gut reaction' as the basis for their selection decisions, or the 'I know one when I see one' approach, leading to expensive mistakes. Despite this, an effective interview remains the most common process in the NHS, mainly because there is still felt to be no substitute for face-to-face discussion with prospective employees.

The effectiveness of the interview can be improved by five factors:

- Mandatory training for panel members in equal opportunities and interview skills – few people are good at intuitive interviewing, most benefit from coaching and better appreciation of the pitfalls.
- Composition of the interview panel – ensuring this is of appropriate seniority, representative of stakeholders in the appointment and knowledgeable about the job requirements.
- Structured interviews based on the person specification – research shows that structured interviews – that is, those which follow a set pattern of questioning – have a higher success rate.

- Objective scoring systems, again based on the person specification.

- Including other appropriate selection tools – for example, presentations, group discussions, written, skill and psychometric tests

Any selection tools used in addition to the interview must be relevant to the job, justifiable, and fair in terms of equality legislation.

Following this process enhances objectivity and provides a robust mechanism for identifying the most suitable candidates. However, it will not in itself protect an organisation against the risk of an unsafe appointment. Processes must be used to establish the credentials of potential employees – as recommended by the reports on Allitt and others.

Credentialling   9.36

It has been estimated that as many as one in eight people exaggerate or falsify their qualifications or other information in their application. In every sector of care it is a first principle to check, at the point of recruitment, that applicants meet the high standards expected by the public.[13] These checks are called 'credentialling', and they establish that the applicant is who they say they are, has the qualifications and references required, and does not have a record of poor performance which would call their suitability into question.

Checks   9.37

For NHS appointments, including volunteers, students and agency workers, the checks [14] are as follows:

- **Qualifications and professional registration** detailed in the application form should be checked with the registration or examination body before employment. Candidates should bring original certificates with them to interview to be checked by the recruitment specialist.

- **Any publications, prizes or awards** detailed in the application should be backed by evidence brought to interview.

- **Proof of identity**, preferably a passport, should be brought to interview. The photograph and information will verify proof of identity, but also serves to check the candidate has the right to live and work in the UK in accordance with the *Immigration and Asylum Act 1996*.

- **Satisfactory references** are needed from the present and most recent employer. Recruiters should validate the identity of referees, and whether they are representative of the person's career history and professional competence.

- **Criminal convictions** should be declared where applicable to the job role and suitability to work with children and vulnerable adults verified.

- **Fitness to practise** –for health professionals NHS employers must obtain a declaration covering any past or pending investigations by a regulatory body.. This must be confirmed at interview, checked and any declarations discussed and considered before a decision on employment is made.

- **Pre-employment health assessment** – applicants should be cleared by occupational health departments.

Good practice for employers is to have a checklist for each candidate, and systems for picking up and dealing with problems. In the NHS this checklist must be kept up to date and incorporate any future national or statutory requirements. Particular note should be taken of the Data Protection Codes of Practice, and of the impact of human rights rulings on employee rights to privacy and access to information in the pre-employment checking process.

Guidance on references   9.38

The purpose of references is to obtain information in confidence from a third party, providing a factual check on a candidate's employment history, qualifications, experience and suitability for the post. References are an essential part of the credentialling process, and must be viewed by appointment panels before a decision on employment is made.

Reliability   9.39

However, it would be misleading to assume that references are always reliable and provide all the information a prospective employer needs. References, like interviews, are one of the most frequently used predictors of candidate suitability, despite research showing validity and reliability problems. References in unstructured letter format can be subjective, telling us more about the referee than about the candidate. In a small number of cases references can also be biased in terms of race or sex, and omit vital information about capability and fitness to practise.

Objectivity and accuracy   9.40

Employers today are more aware of the value of objective references from other employers, particularly in the same healthcare sector. However, they are also aware of recent cases that highlight the dangers of giving inaccurate or misleading references. Negligence claims can arise when facts provided in a reference are not properly checked, and an employer may be in breach of their duty of care to an employee if they fail to confine the reference to factually indisputable statements – for example, by referring to allegations which had not been substantiated.

However, there may also be a breach of the duty of care to other employers if a full and accurate reference is not given. Best guidance is to ensure that a reference, even if factually accurate, does not give an unfair impression of the former employee concerned.

Procedure 9.41

Developing a structured reference form, with forced choice options, and careful scrutiny of referee information can reduce these problems. If the panel does not view references until after the interview, objectivity can also be improved by reducing 'halo effect', particularly if panels also score candidates first. Panels can then see whether references support the ranking. The recruitment specialist should view the references before the interview in case there are issues to be followed up with referees or professional bodies, and of which the interviewers should be aware before they see the candidate.

To protect themselves from negligence or other claims, employers must provide guidance to senior managers on who can provide references and on the content.

Criminal records and protection of the public

Declaration of criminal records 9.42

To safeguard the public, especially children and vulnerable adults, there are exemptions from the *Rehabilitation of Offenders Act 1974* enabling health employers to require applicants for jobs involving direct contact with patients to declare any convictions, whether spent or not under the Act. Employers have well-established procedures to check any declarations at the recruitment stage, and consider whether the nature or timing of the offence makes an applicant unsuitable for the job in question.

It is essential that these procedures are followed. A recent analysis of a sample of job applications found that fewer than 1% of applicants revealed a conviction. This statistic bears no relation to reality, as ex offenders represent up to one third of the working population. According to Home Office statistics, one third of men have been convicted of a crime other than a driving offence by the age of 46.

Statistics also show that most convictions do not result in a custodial sentence, and are for offences other than violence to another person. However, for the healthcare employer, the main concern is to manage the risks of employing an individual, who may gain inappropriate access to children or vulnerable adults.[15]

To reduce the risk of inaccurate or undeclared offences in appropriate roles, recruiters must check that declarations have been completed before shortlisting, and ask applicants to confirm they have no convictions at interview. They must also ask about any gaps in employment, and scrutinise references. If there are offences declared, these must be discussed at interview. Apart from regulated positions, having a criminal record does not necessarily debar an individual from appointment. It is important to ensure that ex offenders are treated fairly, with no unlawful discrimination, and to balance this against the need to protect patients, staff and the public.

Further checks   9.43

More detailed checks must be made on the possible criminal background of potential employees in regulated positions involving the care of children, young persons, or vulnerable adults. The Criminal Records Bureau has been set up to facilitate safer recruitment to protect these groups by making such information more accessible to employers. Health organisations must register with the CRB to obtain enhanced and standard disclosures for appropriate posts to replace the previous system of police checks.

In addition, under the *Protection of Children Act 1999*, childcare organisations must check names against the statutory lists when proposing to appoint someone to a childcare position, to ensure they are not disqualified from such work. Employers must refer names for possible inclusion if an employee harms a child, or puts them at risk of harm, in the course of employment.

Managers must note that they may be committing an offence under the *Criminal Justice and Court Services Act 2000* if they offer work, or allow someone to continue to work in a regulated position, in the knowledge that they are disqualified from such work. It is possible they may also be liable if there are adverse incidents arising from a failure to make appropriate checks.

Review   9.44

The *Rehabilitation of Offenders Act 1974* is over 25 years old, and under review as there are concerns about whether it strikes the right balance between fairness to ex-offenders and the need to protect the public.[16]

Meanwhile, the Criminal Records Bureau advises that recruiters must be fully aware of their duties under all relevant legislation. Ultimately it is the responsibility of the employer to decide whether to offer a job and it is worth remembering that criminal record checks and disclosures are no substitute for thorough pre-employment checks and good interview practice.

Pre-employment occupational health screening   9.45

Pre-employment occupational health screening is an essential risk management element of the recruitment and selection process. This is to facilitate health and safety management, namely:

- identification of people whose health background or personality profile may make them a danger to patients, the public or colleagues;

- identification of existing ill-health which could be aggravated by work duties;

- any adjustments to the duties and responsibilities, or terms and conditions required under the *Disability Discrimination Act 1995*;

- identifying any employees needing follow up referrals; and

- ensuring new employees have the appropriate immunisation status.

Good practice processes in pre-employment health screening include the following:

- Pre-employment health assessment carried out by the occupational health service (OHS) for all healthcare workers.

- Completion of a standard health questionnaire screened by the OHS, with an interview to assess fitness for the post if necessary.

- Details of the applicant's sickness record for the past year – this should be on the personal details/equal opportunities section of the application, seen only by the recruitment specialist to ensure confidentiality. This record should be verified with the previous employer, taking account of guidance from the Information Commissioner on data protection implications.[17]

- The interview should check any absence patterns or discrepancies, and that the applicant does not consider themselves disabled and require adjustments to be considered.

- Obtaining clearance from the occupational health department before an offer of employment is made.

Occupational health service recommendations must be followed to ensure the health and safety of staff, and patients, and to avoid liability.

Extreme cases   9.46

The Clothier report looked at the problem of picking up extreme cases through occupational health clearance because of the difficulty of assessing psychological health, in particular, personality disorder. The report concluded that excessive absence through sickness, excessive use of counselling or medical facilities, and self-harming behaviour are better guides than psychological testing.

From a common-sense point of view, any of these factors are likely to affect competence and performance in past jobs. Careful scrutiny of applications by trained recruiters should identify career or skill gaps and excessive sickness. Good probing questions at interview, covering the technical aspects of the role, past experience and competency scenarios should also identify high-risk people on the basis of failure to meet the person specification.

Avoiding discrimination   9.47

In making decisions on grounds of excessive sickness absence or other health factors, selection panels must be careful not to discriminate against disabled applicants. Unreasonable failure to appoint on grounds of disability is unlawful under the *Disability Discrimination Act 1995*. All NHS employers must now have obtained the Employment Service's Two Ticks disability award, which means any disabled candidate who meets the person specification is offered an interview.

Duty of confidentiality 9.48

Occupational health departments must be provided with a copy of the job description and person specification both to assess adjustments needed in the case of a disability, but also to assess suitability for the job in general. Normally any discussions and outcomes remain confidential, and the manager is only told what is reasonable to be disclosed, but what does an occupational health specialist do if they find a real issue of concern? Should they break confidentiality to the individual, in order to protect patients, fellow professionals and the public generally?

The Bullock report[4] examined the legal and professional code of ethics position in some detail, and concluded that there is no absolute duty of confidentiality. The public interest, as well as the interests of patients, can warrant, in appropriate and justifiable circumstances, disclosure of information. This principle is particularly important when managers refer employees for occupational health assessment because of sickness absence, performance concerns that may be health-related, or other problems arising in the course of employment.

Smart cards 9.49

An initiative that will help speed up health clearance on appointment, for locum doctor appointments and doctors in training, and with the transfer of reliable information between employers, is the NHS occupational health smart card scheme. Smart cards record pre-employment check data, including occupational health and immunisation records. This improvement in portability acknowledges that duplicate checks can be time-consuming for health workers who regularly move within the service – for example, for training – and also potentially costly for employers.

Doctors in training are issued with personalised smart cards containing their name and photograph. All data is securely stored but accessible to authorised personnel at any time. As the card also records data on suitability to work in regulated positions and criminal record checks, recruiters will have immediate information about a doctor's clearance for dealing safely with patients.

Other health issues 9.50

Employers are responsible for ensuring health workers, including locums and agency staff, have the correct immunisation status for the jobs they are to do. Healthcare workers who lack certain immunities may not be able to perform exposure prone clinical procedures. These are procedures where there is a risk that injury to the healthcare worker could result in exposure of the patients open tissues to the blood of the health care worker. This risk arises in invasive surgery, some general practice procedures, obstetrics and gynaecology, dentistry and mid-wifery.

The Department of Health has consulted on action to address the potential health risks posed to patients from new healthcare workers infected with serious communicable diseases, in particular HIV, hepatitis B, hepatitis C and tuberculosis.[18] Anticipated guidance is expected to introduce further health clearance measures for new staff working or training in a clinical care setting.

Where an existing health worker loses immunity or acquires a blood borne virus, their duties may have to be restricted. In this case variations in contracts of employment must be achieved by agreement with the individual, and if termination of employment is the only option, fair processes must be followed to avoid the risk of dismissal claims.

The report on the Elwood case (SEE **9.15**) recommends particular attention to the occupational health assessment of older doctors. Care should be taken not to discriminate against older workers in any systems introduced. A better policy is to ensure clearance is obtained in the same way for all new employees, whether permanent or temporary, and that all employees and managers have access to good occupational health advice during employment.

External recruitment services   9.51

There are three main ways in which external recruitment services are used in healthcare:

- to provide specialist temporary workers on a regular basis (mainly nurses and locum doctors);

- to obtain short-term cover where internal solutions are not available (mainly administrative and clerical staff); and

- for executive search in key or hard-to-fill senior posts (for example, chief executives or medical directors).

Staff shortages and an increasing preference from workers for the more flexible employment arrangements agency work can offer, means agencies are playing an increasing role in shaping the healthcare workforce. Many employers have come to rely on external agencies to meet their staffing needs.

Agencies' obligations   9.52

The present law sets out minimum standards of conduct for employment agencies: agencies should check workers have the qualifications required by law for the job they are to do, and should obtain enough information to show a worker is suitable for the job. Higher standards to protect the public are being introduced including better checking of qualifications to ensure workers are not sent to do work which puts their and others' health and safety at risk because it is outside their experience or competence. Agencies will have to obtain references where temporary workers will be in regulated positions with children or vulnerable adults.

Many health employers already require this of agencies in service specifications. However, in practice experience shows reliance on this is not enough and employers must make their own checks. Incidents may not have been reported, and may only come to light through enquiries of previous employers. Good practice is to carry out appropriate pre-employment checks in the same way as you would for permanent staff.

Casual worker banks   9.53

Many acute trusts have tried to overcome this problem (and also cut costs in agency fees) by establishing their own casual worker banks, particularly for nurses, administrative and secretarial staff. This enables employers to check qualifications, registration and previous experience when people first join the bank, and to keep track of their capability. However bank staff, like agency workers, often do not have access to training and are not able to keep their skills up to date in the same way as permanent staff, and the casual nature of their employment means their contribution to the workforce is not maximised.

NHS Professionals   9.54

NHS Professionals, a programme that aims to combine the flexibility of agency and bank work with the benefits and perceived greater safety of NHS employment, is being rolled out across the NHS in nursing and medical specialties.

Probationary contracts   9.55

Probationary periods of employment are often used in the health service where an occupational health review is required, but their main value is to enable an employer to assess whether a new employee is truly suitable for the job. This is especially valuable for clinical governance and assuring the quality of care, but there are pitfalls to be avoided in making appointments on a probationary basis.

Legal pitfalls   9.56

The pitfalls are partly legal – for example, failing to make it clear that employment is not guaranteed for the probationary period, but may be terminated by notice. If there is a need to terminate a contract before the end of the probationary period, then notice and operation of any disciplinary procedures must be in accordance with the contract. To avoid extending employment unnecessarily, notice periods while on probation should be shorter than for permanent employees, and there should be a shorter, less complex disciplinary procedure.

Managerial pitfalls   9.57

The other pitfalls are managerial: there is no point in having a probationary period if managers fail to monitor an employee's progress and to take action if it is not satisfactory, as once the probationary period expires it becomes a permanent contract. Probationary periods are generally three or six months, which is often not long enough to assess an individual, particularly in a complex role. They may also affect recruitment, as people in permanent jobs take a risk when accepting posts which are subject to satisfactory completion of a probationary period.

For all these reasons, probationary contracts are not widely used in NHS organisations, and employers rely on monitoring and action to improve performance, followed by normal capability or disciplinary procedures and appeal arrangements if the progress of a new employee is not satisfactory. Care must, however, be taken to initiate any action promptly, as delay in operating procedures may mean that employees have built up the one-year qualifying period for complaint to an employment tribunal. Ideally, procedures must always be operated fully and fairly, even if the employee has less than one year's service, as complaints may still be brought on grounds of sex, race, disability, and other discrimination grounds, together with pregnancy, maternity, trade union membership or certain aspects of industrial action, without the need for a qualifying period of employment.

Induction training programmes   9.58

There has been increasing recognition of the importance of induction courses and the initial settling-in period for employee retention, motivation and embedding safe working practices. Considerable time and effort is devoted to recruitment and selection processes. An unsuccessful appointment, can affect corporate momentum, as well as increase costs and personal distress.[19]

The employee is one of the variables in the risk management monitoring model. Induction is one way of raising employee awareness of how they can influence quality and make a real difference to the management of risk.

The way in which employees are received into an organisation is a crucial factor in forming their attitudes and ensuring they reach the required high standard of performance. This is the time when cultural issues, like the importance of teamworking and respect for patients raised in the Bristol inquiry, can be reinforced, and the risks associated with care provision reduced.

Corporate induction   9.59

Good practice is to have a corporate induction programme attended by all new employees within two months of starting work. A typical programme might include:

- introduction by the chief executive;
- key issues for the organisation;
- mission, values and standards;
- human resource policies;
- health and safety; and
- fire and emergency procedures.

Key issues discussed can include human resource areas identified by risk management assessment, for example pre-employment checks or appraisal.

Local induction   9.60

In addition, managers must develop local induction programmes to meet the needs of new employees in the work area. The main benefits of this approach are:

- New employees settle in quickly and become productive early.
- Motivation is increased and maintained.
- Employee turnover, lateness, absenteeism and poor performance may be reduced.
- It helps to develop a management style where the emphasis is on leadership.
- Employees work in a safer environment.

Time with line managers   9.61

It is important that new employees meet and spend time with their colleagues in the first days and understand the culture. Research suggests that, when employees leave a job early, most cited getting on with the boss as a crucial factor. It is important to arrange quality time with the line manager, when standards and responsibility can be reinforced, as this is where most problems are likely to occur.

Disaffected people are probably also those who may give rise to risk – for example, from failure to follow procedures fully or to the best of their ability.

Organisations must have a checklist of items for managers to go through with new staff on their first day. Typically these include: terms and conditions of employment, duties and responsibilities, standards and rules of conduct, health and safety, and confidentiality. In a busy department, with staff shortages, it is easy to skimp on local, initial induction. This is poor practice, providing another example of how short cuts can open up risk for the organisation.

The NHS places particular importance on induction for newly qualified medical and dental staff and for doctors joining another hospital or moving to another speciality. Induction courses are compulsory for pre-registration posts and must cover management issues, professional concerns such as death certification, breaking bad news, and keeping GPs informed of their patients' progress.

Addressing poor clinical performance   9.62

The NHS consultation document *Supporting doctors, protecting patients*[20] on preventing, recognising and dealing with poor clinical performance of doctors was published in response to a number of recent inquiries, particularly Bristol, and public concern. Acknowledging the need for change, the document also pictures success, stating that over the past decade the demands on doctors have changed substantially. These include workload pressures, higher public and patient expectations, advances in technology, new responsibilities to meet explicit clinical standards and greater emphasis on training. The document states: 'Doctors have shown remarkable ability to rise to these challenges and, year after year, the majority deliver a first-class service to their patients.'

Key lessons   9.63

The number of cases of poor clinical performance hitting the headlines has important lessons for skill updating, which are just as applicable to non-clinical staff. Key lessons for effective clinical governance systems include:

* Although many cases were presented as a single incident, when investigated it was clear that a pattern of poor practice had developed over a long period of time.

* Although such problems may not have been officially recognised, they were often known about in informal networks.

* Systems that might have been expected to detect poor outcomes of care and weak processes had failed to pick up problems with the practice of the doctor concerned.

The document cites in particular the Bristol inquiry and the further case of a gynaecologist dismissed by South Kent Hospitals NHS Trust in early 1996 because of apparent serious failures in clinical practice.

Unsatisfactory disciplinary procedures   9.64

The human resource function has a key role where suspension and dismissal is concerned, but medical disciplinary procedures do not adequately cover the need to involve the human resources function at an early stage for professional employment advice. As a result, procedures do not provide proper protection for patients, are cumbersome and costly to operate, and are not always fair to doctors.

New national procedures covering medical staff are being developed, but meanwhile what are the remedial and educational solutions recommended and currently being put in place by health employers?

Continuing professional development (CPD)   9.65

CPD programmes are the means by which healthcare professionals and managers ensure their knowledge and skills are up to date. As an example, in future all doctors will have to show evidence of personal development plans and action on CPD as part of the appraisal process operated by employers and for revalidation by the General Medical Council (GMC).

Human resource practitioners have a key role in the introduction of CPD for doctors in their organisation, and in the employment issues when remedial training or other action is needed. While remedial training is ongoing, human resource practitioners will have to resolve alternative employment, job plan revisions and adjustments to contracts of employment, in consultation with clinical directors, individual doctors and their staff representative.

Appraisal   9.66

Appraisal has been a feature of managing senior and administrative health workers for some time, but as several of the reports found, is less embedded for clinicians.

The NHS Plan announced the intention that all doctors employed or under contract to the NHS will, as a condition of contract, be required to participate in annual appraisal from 2001. Appraisal is defined[20] as a positive process to give feedback on performance, chart continuing progress and identify development needs. It is a forward-looking process essential for the developmental and educational planning needs of an individual.

Individual responsibility for risk   9.67

However, to address risk, the appraisal and personal development plan process must include an assessment of individual responsibility for risk. This should be based on quantitative and qualitative data on performance, and identify the lessons learned from errors or untoward outcomes.

As an example, the consultant appraisal scheme is described as a professional process of constructive dialogue, in which the doctor being appraised has a formal structured opportunity to reflect on their work and consider how their performance might be improved. The scheme content focuses on clinical aspects of the consultant's work, including audit activity reports, any investigations following complaints, risk management, professional relationships with patients and colleagues, and teamworking.

The problem for the human resource professional and the manager is to make sure all this happens; that comprehensive annual appraisals do take place and that outcomes are realistic and pursued.

To this extent, the problems of appraisal for consultants are no different to those for other health workers; there is an equal need for appraisal in the case of nurses (as shown by the Clothier and Bullock reports) and other health professionals and managers, as there is for the most junior administrative and clerical staff. Good appraisal will have an impact on quality of care and reduction of risk.

Regulation and revalidation   9.68

The current medical regulation system determines who should enter and remain in the profession at different levels and in different fields of practice, helping organisations achieve high quality standards through clinical governance. Protection of the public demands that entry to the professional registers should be on the basis of reliable and vital evidence of capability to practice. The General Medical Council is currently considering new criteria which will mean that procedures for entry to the Medical Register include not just the knowledge, skills and experience necessary for medical practice, but also probity, health and conduct.[21]

The GMC is also introducing a revalidation process that will require all doctors to demonstrate on a regular basis that they continue to be fit to practice. Revalidation will be linked to NHS appraisal schemes.

Referrals   9.69

Employers have a public duty, to report serious problems to the GMC independently of any disciplinary or other action taken by the employer. This is particularly important if the doctor is dismissed and is likely to practice elsewhere, as the GMC is the only body which can suspend or remove a doctor's registration. Referrals should also be made where there is evidence of false claims regarding qualifications, experience or publications. The employer should also consider informing other employers through the national alert letter system.[22]

The position here is no different to other health professionals. The issue for human resource specialists is to ensure proper, prompt procedures for dealing with poor practice or inappropriate behaviour and determining whether a referral to the regulatory body should be made. Referral should only be made where an initial prompt investigation provides accurate, documented evidence of a case to answer. Special care must be taken to ensure there is no discrimination on grounds of race, sex, disability, or other unlawful grounds, and that confidentiality is observed.

Retraining in the light of lessons from incidents   9.70

Understanding how risk arises, and the consequences of working where risk may arise, is a learning process. Organisations must understand the causes of risk, and its link with quality.

Learning from people management failures, adverse incidents and near-misses in organisations is very important for organisational development and business success. John Peters, the Gulf War veteran, says in an article in the journal *People Management*:

> 'Individual trial and error is a very ineffective way to learn. It is infinitely better to learn from someone else's mistakes rather than your own. If companies can create an open culture where people feel safe admitting their mistakes, then corporate wisdom will grow dramatically.'[23]

The Health and Safety Executive (HSE), found a high number of employers do not have proper procedures in place for assessing the causes of accidents and learning from them.[24] In the NHS, there is now a single national system of reporting adverse patient events and near-misses through the National Patient Safety Agency (NPSA).

As well as making sure events are reported in the first place, the NPSA aims to promote an open and fair culture in the NHS, encouraging all healthcare staff to report incidents without fear of personal recrimination. The intention is that the information provided will help identify patterns and key underlying factors to establish patient safety priorities. These solutions will be fed back to staff and organisations.

OWAM recommendations   9.71

The DOH report *An Organisation with a Memory* (see **KEY REFERENCES, APPENDIX 1**) addresses the need for a national system to identify and learn effectively from incidents. It advocates a change in culture towards reporting by encouraging more open and blame-free approaches, to ensure that lessons learnt in one part of the organisation are properly shared with the whole.

The main human resources recommendations from this report are the need for:

- a more open culture, in which errors or service failures can be reported and discussed; and

- mechanisms for ensuring that, where lessons are identified, the necessary changes are put into practice.

Learning from incidents and complaints needs to be an integral feature of appraisal systems, with individual retraining needs identified and incorporated in personal development plans. Where learning from incidents indicates a wider organisational need, the required changes must be incorporated in induction programmes, education and training courses. This is particularly relevant to cultural issues. Other lessons are the need for more effective training management, teambuilding and leadership.

Leadership and management development   9.72

All healthcare organisations should have leadership development plans in place which focus on personal leadership qualities, and those needed for improving clinical quality and leading modernisation programmes. Nationally, this is being rolled out through the NHS Leadership Centre programme.

Understanding risk   9.73

Part of improving clinical quality is reducing the adverse effect of risk. Leadership is important for risk management, in terms of ensuring a well-run organisation with high care standards, but also to develop risk management as a concept within the organisation, providing a constant reminder of its value and of the consequences of not taking account of risk.

Similarly, management training programmes, which include decision-making, must consider the consequences of individual judgments and the impact on risk. In people management, poor judgment often arises when established systems or routines are ignored or manipulated, often for short-term gain. Management development programmes must therefore include consideration of the rationale for a systems approach to high-risk areas, and an understanding of the flexibilities available, as well as the processes for introducing change. They must also include educating managers to be able to identify, assess and control risks.

Senior management development   9.74

All healthcare organisations should also have management training strategies, which take on board the lessons from adverse incidents. Human resource professionals can have a key role in brokering senior management/board level development by:

- advising on development opportunities; and

- facilitating the arrangements – for example, by study leave policies or cover for the job.

Useful approaches to senior management development include:

- outside organisation options – secondments, development programmes, academic courses;

- mentoring, coaching and shadowing;

- learning groups;
- 360-degree feedback (from colleagues, subordinates and managers); and
- e-learning.

Creating a learning organisation, where training needs at all levels, including senior managers and professionals, are addressed, is essential for benefiting from mistakes or near-misses and poor practice.

Code of conduct for NHS Managers 9.75

As part of the response to the Kennedy report, a code of practice[25] for NHS managers has been produced. This sets out the core standards of conduct expected of NHS managers and aims to contribute to reassuring the public that local decisions are made against a background of professional standards and accountability.

Central to the code is that NHS management calls for difficult decisions and complicated choices, and the interests of staff and patients may not always coincide. The code applies to all managers, and must be incorporated in contracts of employment.

High-performance, patient-centred teams 9.76

There is increasing recognition that high-quality patient-centred care relies upon effective teamworking across traditional skill groups and staff boundaries. Where staff work in teams, they work more effectively. Recent research[26] shows a strong link between high levels of team working, and reduced patient mortality.

Features of effective teams were found to be:

- Shared objectives.
- Interdependent working.
- Interaction and information sharing.
- Task emphasis.
- Clear roles.
- Recognition as a team.

The research suggests that if more staff worked as teams, patient mortality will be reduced even further. Leadership in teams also has an effect: a lack of clear leadership was associated with high levels of stress among team members.

The research also found that if diverse professional groups (for example, general practitioners, primary care nurses, physiotherapists, counsellors) work well together, there are better quality decisions about patient care, and more innovations in patient care. The same was found for breast cancer care teams.

Why do teams fail?

In summary, teams fail where there is a lack of:

- mutual respect, trust and openness;
- clarity on respective roles; and
- clear leadership.

Teambuilding exercises with an external facilitator can help address these problems.

Team bonus pilots 9.77

In the NHS, team bonus schemes are being introduced to identify the most effective ways of rewarding and incentivising high-quality performance. These schemes aim to test how far team based rewards help to:

- clarify goals and priorities at team and organisational level; and
- encourage cooperative work and behaviour.

The premise is that individual bonuses can be divisive, while team bonuses can strengthen links between colleagues and encourage more collaborative work.

Early reported outcomes from team bonus schemes include improvements to patient choice in non – emergency appointment times, and improvements to patient pathways, for example, admission via Emergency Assessment Units and same day diagnostic services.

Importance of adequate resources 9.78

In managing risk, it has to be accepted that additional resources may be needed. One of the present main areas of concern is the effect of staffing shortages on maintenance and development of services.

Staff shortages 9.79

The report on the Bristol inquiry says that the inquiry team was 'sometimes amazed' that the paediatric cardiac service could be maintained at all, such was the staff shortage. Specialist cardiologists and surgeons were found to be below a proper level and lacked junior support. According to the report, understaffing was so great that the cardiologists could not participate effectively in surgery or intensive care. There was a shortage of nurses trained in care of children, theatre work and intensive care.

The NHS Plan recognises that the biggest constraints facing the delivery of healthcare today are around workforce shortages, and many feel that the only way the modernisation agenda and patient-centred care will be delivered is by greater investment in frontline staff. The Plan proposes increases in the number of consultants, GPs and nurses, but it will take several years before resource investment pays off.

Initiatives to increase numbers 9.80

There are a number of initiatives in hand to increase numbers in the short term. One is the national advertising campaign to encourage trained nurses and other healthcare professionals who have left to return. Flexible working, nursery provision and return-to-practice refresher courses and assigned mentors have been successful in recruiting many former employees.

Under the NHS Professionals programme, nurses can work shift patterns that suit them and are supported by training and skill updating. Self-rostering arrangements have had considerable success in boosting staff availability for work and contributing to adequate resourcing.

International recruitment 9.81

International recruitment is another major central strategy. Looking globally to resolve home skill shortages makes business sense, but raises ethical issues about the impact on home and developing country labour markets and economies. The NHS agreed in 1999 that it would not recruit from countries that were themselves facing shortages of health professionals, especially poorer nations. International nurse recruitment has therefore been targeted at countries where there is a recognised surplus of health staff.

There are risks involved. Candidates appointed must have similar skills and competences to staff trained in the UK. Nurses arriving in the UK attend courses to improve their English and their knowledge of UK health systems of care, and provide advice on issues such as setting up bank accounts and finding accommodation. Expert teams trained in credentialling professionals from other countries are needed to recruit them.

The Government is now looking to recruit consultants and GPs from countries such as Spain that have a doctor surplus.[27] but is imperative that doctors coming to work in the UK are offered structured induction programmes and support to enable them to settle into practice in order to reduce clinical governance risks.

Balanced skill mix 9.82

Having the right skill mix in the workforce is important in healthcare. This is primarily for cost reasons – healthcare is labour intensive and people account for a high proportion of total costs. Second, it is important for quality improvement, which in turn reduces the risk of errors. In a time of skill shortage, changes to skill

251

mix, and the development of a more flexibly skilled workforce is crucial for achieving improvements in clinical practice.

What is meant by skill mix? There are variations in definition. The term can refer to the mix of posts in the establishment, the mix of employees in a post, the combination of skills available at a specific time, or, alternatively, it may refer to the combination of activities in each role.[28]

For the NHS, interest in skill mix is partly prompted by the need to fill the gap caused by a shortage in supply of staff. The approach to skill mix review here is to explore alternative staffing solutions, such as redesigning roles or skill substitution. However skill mix review is increasingly prompted by new approaches to care, such as patient-focused care, partnership working with social services departments, the independent and voluntary sectors, and developments in primary care.

Alternative staffing solutions   9.83

Expanding the role of nurses to use their skills and experience in tasks traditionally carried out by doctors was set out as a key objective in the NHS Plan. Specialist nurses in NHS trusts now book patients into their own operating lists and carry out minor operations. In orthopaedics, for example, this can reduce waiting times for patients with minor conditions.

Specialist GPs are also starting to carry out minor surgery and diagnostic procedures to speed up waiting times for their patients and release pressure on local hospitals. They can filter out cases they can deal with, and make sure a consultant sees urgent or complicated cases.

The need for greater consultant-led services – for example, 24-hour cover in labour wards – means redesigning services and the mix of staff and roles in the teams providing the service. Teams in obstetrics can include a mix of specialist consultants, staff grade doctors, senior house officers or specialist registrars, and nurse or midwife practitioners. This offers better training for doctors and continuity of expert care for patients.

The Changing Workforce Programme is a national programme helping health and social care organisations to develop new ways of working to improve patient services, tackle staff shortages and increase job satisfaction. The programme includes a national database of new job roles, for organisations to take on board. An example of these new roles is physician's assistants, who can provide a rapid assessment of medical patients, which may reduce admissions.

NHS Direct   9.84

NHS Direct is a further example of using resources differently, allowing front line staff to work more effectively. Routing telephone calls from accident and emergency departments to NHS Direct mean nurses can now spend more time with patients.

Staff retention   9.85

Staff retention is another essential feature of adequate resourcing for the modernisation programme and safe systems of care. Many qualified staff leave to work abroad, or for family or other personal reasons. Failing to keep staff can be costly in terms of replacement, but the organisation also loses valuable skills, knowledge and experience, often gained by years of expensive training. In some medical specialties this is currently irreplaceable.

There continues to be concern about attrition from NHS funded pre- registration healthcare courses. An estimated 20% of nursing students, and up to18% of allied health professional students fail to complete their training programme. These attrition rates are not dissimilar to other higher education courses, but represent wasted resources. Work is being done to better identify the reasons why NHS students join, drop out or transfer from programmes. Modular courses enabling students to step on and off programmes is one way forward.[29]

Boosting retention – pay and HR policies

Pay and reward   9.86

So how can an employer boost retention? Good induction, is invaluable. Paying the going rate is also important – financial packages must be fair and motivating, based on pay market data and job evaluation. Modernising pay and rewards is progressing through the *Agenda for change* initiative. This is built on the premise that it is important to have pay arrangements that reward staff for the work they do, and the skills and competencies they develop, providing a firm basis for improving the quality of care. *Agenda for change* is underpinned by key tools: a new job evaluation scheme and a Knowledge and Skills Framework, which aims to provide a better means of recognising the skills and knowledge needed to be effective in a particular role (see also **CHAPTER 3**).

Pay can be a key retention issue, a 'psychological last straw' if people are demoralised, or feel they cannot really make a difference in the organisation. An example is when NHS employees see agency workers earning more than them for perceived less responsibility.

HR policies   9.87

Good human resource policies have a role in making people feel valued by providing a framework for employees to work within and understand what is expected of them. Essential core policies are discipline and grievance, health and safety, trade union recognition and consultation. However, training opportunities and flexible working, are just as important for retention. Human resource strategy must include personal development plans for each employee, balancing the needs of the organisation with a rewarding role for individuals and a real improvement to their working lives.

Flexible working   9.88

The NHS Improving Working Lives Standard recognises the value of a well-managed, flexible working environment that supports staff, promotes their welfare and development and provides a productive work-life balance. In a predominantly female workforce, having a range of family-friendly policies can also boost retention. The good healthcare employer will have in place policies on flexible working, such as part-time working, jobsharing and homeworking, special and carer leave, maternity, paternity and parental leave, nursery and out-of-school care places. For working parents, the right to request flexible working and the duty of the employer to consider that request is now statutory under the *Employment Act 2002*. Part-time workers are also protected under the *Part–time Workers (Prevention of less favourable treatment) Regulations 2000 (SI 2000/2035)*.

Morale   9.89

Media headlines often refer to low morale in organisations and the impact on safety. In healthcare, low morale is attributed to many factors including high stress levels, racism, poor staffing levels and working conditions. Low morale is one of the reasons why people leave their jobs. Investing in staff can boost productivity by increasing morale and lowering staff turnover, and can also improve patient satisfaction.

Measuring and improving morale   9.90

Improving and sustaining staff morale is another key factor in the national strategy for achieving high quality patient centered services, and reducing risk. Morale can be defined as the confidence, enthusiasm and discipline of a person or group at a particular time. So how can morale be properly gauged, and what sort of staff investment will make a difference? Use of annual staff attitude surveys enables employers to identify the things employees think they do well, and those which require improvement. This tool can help measure progress in improving the quality of working life for staff. Further action in the areas identified can in turn improve retention, motivation and quality of care.

Two areas employers are increasingly looking to invest in, with the aim of directly impacting on morale and motivation, are communications and staff involvement.

Employee communication   9.91

Employee communication is well recognised as an important action area in times of restructuring, mergers or cost reduction. Organisational morale can be particularly low when people are waiting to hear how jobs will be filled in the new organisation, who will be transferred and which jobs may no longer be required. As well as maintaining work levels during times of turbulence, employers are anxious to retain skills during the transition. In the case of most healthcare roles, these are key skill areas that will be needed in the new organisation.

Communication strategies are also important for projecting key messages about risk management and good practice in patient care. Morale can improve if staff feel they are working for an effective and well respected organisation. To this extent, publicising success (new ways of working or of improving patient choice or satisfaction, for example) has been shown to contribute to improved performance ratings.

All health organisations should have an employee communications strategy setting out how people will be kept up to date with key developments and able to input their own views and questions. Communication mechanisms include:

- Face-to-face dialogue – small or large groups, and an open door policy.

- Mechanisms for structured feedback from employees and evidence that this is listened to, for example, working and focus groups, question and answer sheets.

- Briefings – organisational and team, by Email, notice boards and other communication systems.

- Training and awareness raising.

- Websites.

- Distribution of letters, memos, meeting notes, annual reports.

- Newsletters, bulletins, news sheets.

- Telephone help lines, confidential counselling service.

These methods need to be evaluated to decide which types are most effective for the message to be conveyed.

Staff involvement   9.92

Good communication up, down and across the organisation is one of the key outcomes of a staff involvement strategy. An involving, open culture, where everyone understands the organisation's goals, is an important part of fostering a sense of belonging and raising standards. Staff involvement, including partnership working with trade unions, networks and working groups, to enable staff to participate in care practice development, and organisational development are also important.

Sickness absence   9.93

High sickness absence in an organisation is another factor hindering strategies for adequate resourcing. Absence rates vary between different types of health professionals, but sickness absence has the same effect of depriving teams of key skills which often have to be covered at short notice by locum, bank or agency staff.

The cost of sickness absence is currently estimated as £567 per employee per year.[30] UK workers take an average nine days sickness absence per year, mostly short spells of minor illness, and the rate is higher in the public than private sector. Many employers believe that around one-third of absence is not due to actual ill-health and that there is significant under reporting of time off.

Effective sickness absence policies 9.94

It goes without saying therefore that health employers can make considerable cost savings, and improve the quality of healthcare, by effective sickness absence policies. Effective management of the health and welfare of people at work can contribute to performance improvement as well as lowering absenteeism, improving morale and reducing litigation costs associated with ill-health and industrial injuries. Family-friendly and flexible working policies are also important for providing the means for people to manage childcare and other domestic crises without 'going sick'.

The features of an effective sickness absence policy include:

• monitoring of absence by managers, with triggers for investigation;

• return to work interviews with managers to identify poor attendance and occupational causes;

• mechanisms for referral to occupational health services;

• fair processes for dealing with persistent short-term absence; and

• procedures for handling alternative employment, rehabilitation and, if necessary, capability dismissals due to long-term ill-health.

Rehabiliation and disability 9.95

All aspects of the procedure must comply with the provisions of the *Disability Discrimination Act 1995*. Where action is being taken concerning employees whose illness or condition brings them within the scope of the Act, the employer will have to show that it has not discriminated against the employee as a result of their disability. It is essential in cases of long-term ill-health to offer any alternative employment that the employee can do, making reasonable adjustments in accordance with the Act, and case managing rehabilitation back to work.

Stress at work 9.96

Stress is one of the most frequent causes of sickness absence at work, aggravated in healthcare by staff shortages, violence against staff and the demands of their roles. Occupational stress poses a risk to all businesses, illustrated by a number of high profile cases of claims for damages caused by work-related stress. The HSE considers occupational stress to be the second most common work-related illness after back pain.

As discussed in CHAPTER 6, employers have a general duty under health and safety legislation to undertake risk assessments and manage activities to reduce the risk to employees from stress in their jobs. To comply with legal requirements and avoid the risks of claims, , health employers must have stress management policies in place, and systems for risk assessment of work related stress.

In 2003, the first HSE improvement notice in relation to stress was served on Dorset General Hospitals NHS Trust. This arose from complaints from former and current employees of the hospital of intolerably high stress levels at work, caused by staff shortages and long working hours. The HSE concluded that the Trust had inadequate procedures to assess the risk of stress to staff.

It is generally believed that only a sustainable stress management programme will fully protect against claims, and detect incidents of stress. Such a programme should include:

- Risk assessment.
- Audit of HR systems, for example the way grievances or claims of bullying are handled.
- Review of records.
- Employee assistance programmes.
- Family friendly policies.
- Follow up action.

These should help identify the causes .of stress, aim to minimise them and provide employees with a counselling service for confidential advice and support.

Counselling 9.97

Health organisations are increasingly realising the value of employee assistance, or counselling services. In an environment where jobs are stressful, confidential and independent helpline services can support employees and provide them with access to the specialist advice they need to enable them to carry on with their roles. This process helps employees to understand the risks to their own and others' safety, the possible consequences of those risks and how they can be minimised. Human resource policies aimed at avoiding violence at work for frontline staff – for example, ambulance and accident and emergency workers – address this.

Personal problems 9.98

Counselling, or employee assistance programmes, can also help people cope with personal problems, which may be affecting them at work as well as at home, and contribute to risk. These problems may include alcohol or drug abuse, relationship difficulties, ageing parents or financial worries. All employers should have human resource policies that enable them to deal sympathetically with employees with drug and alcohol problems, including referral to occupational health services, but that also manage the risk to patients and fellow workers.

Dealing with distress   9.99

Health organisations, particularly the emergency services, are in the frontline in major accidents and disaster scenarios. While teams of professionals are trained to deal with distressing situations, many emergency workers will still need access to counselling services to cope with their reactions. Employers who provide these are more likely to retain key staff, enable them to continue effectively in their specialist roles, and to manage the risks they face, or must make decisions about, every day.

Distress can be particularly triggered by cases of violence or aggression against healthcare staff. Health organisations must have policies in accordance with the *Zero Tolerance* campaign to deal with offenders, and to report on different types of violence and aggression, including verbal abuse and physical assault.

People management of non-clinical staff   9.100

NHS national guidance reinforces the need for human resource policies and strategy to support clinical governance and performance improvement.

> 'We have always recognised that offering fast, quality care to patients and delivering modern and dependable services with courtesy and understanding means attracting and retaining high quality staff, committed to developing their skills and keeping them up to date.'[31]

This applies as much to non-clinical health workers, or other health professionals as to clinicians. Although most of the examples given so far in this chapter concern medical or nursing staff, it is worth remembering that a large proportion of health workers are non-clinical, including ancillary, scientific and technical, ambulance, administrative and clerical staff and senior managers. Many of the good practice processes described apply equally to them, as there are many non-clinical workers with access to patients or equipment, where risks may arise.

Better regulation   9.101

The Health Professionals Council is the statutory regulatory body which sets and maintains professional standards for healthcare professions, including paramedics, art therapists, podiatrists, clinical scientists, dieticians, medical laboratory technicians, occupational therapists, radiographers and physiotherapists. Its role is to:

- Set standards of proficiency and training.
- Keep a register of those fit to practise.
- Deal with failures to meet the standards.

Health employers must ensure relevant staff are registered with the Council. Otherwise they could be compromising patient safety and the organisation's risk management strategy.

Operating Department Practitioners– a case study   9.102

Action to raise standards and manage risk is seen in the example of operating department practitioners (ODPs – formerly known as theatre technicians). Their professional association holds and maintains a register of operating department practitioners, with the aims of protecting the public and ensuring that all registered ODPs conform to a code of professional conduct and are fit to practise. There is a formal structure for dealing with complaints about conduct, and all health employers must now check with the register before employing ODPs.

Recruitment and selection   9.103

For all employees, it is important to carry out pre-employment checks, thorough induction, training and appraisal, and to learn from errors and risks. Although for many jobs there will not be a direct impact on patient care, there will almost certainly be an indirect effect. This can be seen, potentially, in failures to order equipment, to manage finances, or to route emergency calls correctly, for example.

Managers carry out most NHS recruitment and selection, although professionals are often involved in the process. Many managers in this role do not realise that they may have a personal liability for any adverse incidents resulting from failure to carry out pre-employment checks correctly, as well as the potential to involve their employer in risk and damage to public confidence. This is seen in the criticism of recruiters in several of the major reports.

The impact of under-investment in people   9.104

Healthcare organisations are highly complex, and weak links can have significant impact on frontline services – the effect, often, of shortcuts or under-investment in areas where a real difference can be made. An example of this is the current drive to improve ward cleanliness, a subject of frequent public criticism and a perceived measure of healthcare standards. Under-investment in the management and delivery of cleaning services is now being addressed, and seen as a key performance indicator for NHS trusts. Yet poor performance of individuals, high sickness absence and labour turnover can just as easily jeopardise this initiative and affect delivery of clinical services.

Similarly, in several pilot schemes, clerical and administrative workers are at the forefront of new hospital booking systems allowing patients to choose a date for their first appointment. Admissions booked in this way maximises slots available and can shorten waiting lists because patients are more likely to keep an appointment which suits them. This can have a positive impact on the productivity of frontline staff, but again can be jeopardised just as easily by poor people management.

New roles and policies   9.105

Family-friendly policies, training, particularly in information technology and computing, and good recruitment practice can equally enhance the efficiency and motivation of clerical staff in these kinds of roles. New roles are being created to reinforce this process of increasing people's contribution in the workplace. Childcare coordinators have a direct impact on sickness absence by helping staff find high quality, reliable childcare.

The NHS human resource performance framework introduces performance measures for employers to achieve in these areas, reiterating that the demonstration of how standards are met is increasingly seen as the way forward.

Discrimination and other claims   9.106

The statutory framework relevant to risk management is not confined to health and safety but includes other areas of employment law.

This chapter includes several references to risks arising from a failure to prevent unlawful discrimination. Current UK legislation covers discrimination on grounds of sex, race, and disability and gender reassignment, and from December 2003, religion or belief and sexual orientation in the workplace. Discrimination is a developing area of law, and employers must keep up to date on case law developments.

Sex discrimination   9.107

The *Sex Discrimination Act 1975* (*SDA 1975*) prohibits sex discrimination against individuals in the areas of employment, education and the provision of goods, facilities and services. It also prohibits discrimination in employment against married people.

The *SDA 1975* prohibits both direct and indirect discrimination. Direct discrimination is where a woman (or a man) is treated less favourably than a person of the opposite sex in comparable circumstances is, or would be, because of their sex. Types of direct discrimination include refusal to offer a job on the grounds of an individual's sex, sexual harassment and treating a woman adversely because she is pregnant.

Indirect discrimination is where a condition or practice is applied to both sexes but it adversely affects a larger proportion of one sex than the other, and it is not justifiable, irrespective of sex, to apply that condition or practice. Indirect discrimination may arise in employment for example in connection with shift change proposals, restrictions in hours of work, refusal to allow job sharing, and age and height restrictions in job descriptions.

Gender reassignment   9.108

The *Sex Discrimination (Gender Reassignment) Regulations 1999 (SI 1999/1102)* prohibit direct discrimination on grounds of gender reassignment in employment and vocational training. This covers less favourable treatment on the grounds that an individual intends to undergo, is undergoing, or has undergone, gender reassignment. Health employers need to have policies covering staff and gender reassignment.

Race and ethnic origin   9.109

The *Race Relations Act 1976* provides protection from race discrimination in employment, education, training, housing and the provision of goods, facilities and services. Direct discrimination is when someone is treated less favourably on grounds of his or her colour, race, nationality or national or ethnic origin, than others in similar circumstances. Examples are racist abuse and harassment. Indirect discrimination occurs when people from a racial group are less likely to be able to comply with a requirement or condition, which applies to everyone, but which cannot be justified other than on racial grounds.

Note that the *Race Relations Act 1976 (Amendment) Regulations 2003 (SI 2003/1626)* brought in a new definition of indirect discrimination relating to the application of a provision, criterion or practice on grounds of race or ethnic or national origin. This follows implementation of the EU Race Discrimination Directive, and the original legislation continues to apply to complaints on grounds of colour or nationality. This is likely to cause some confusion on individual rights in the short term, and employers are advised to seek specialist HR advice.

The *Race Relations (Amendment) Act 2000* prohibits race discrimination in all public functions. Public bodies, including health authorities and trusts, have a statutory general duty to promote race equality in all they do, and to produce annual race equality schemes.

Disability   9.110

The *Disability Discrimination Act 1995 (DDA)* makes it unlawful for employers to treat a disabled person less favourably on the grounds of disability, without a justifiable reason. The *DDA 1995* covers recruitment, selection and promotion, and recently has also been held to include selection for redundancy. Capability dismissal on grounds of ill-health will also probably be caught by the *DDA 1995*, and fair procedures, including offers of alternative employment, must be followed.

To come under the protection of the *DDA 1995*, a person must have a disability. This is defined as a physical or mental impairment, causing substantial and long-term effect on ability to carry out day-to-day activities. These definitions are being increasingly clarified by case law, and employers must ensure their corporate knowledge is kept up to date.

For guidance on the employer's duty to make reasonable adjustments in relation to a disabled person see the *Disability Rights Commission Code of Practice – Employment and Occupation* (currently in draft form).

Religion and belief 9.111

Under the *Employment Equality (Religion or Belief) Regulations 2003 (SI 2003/1660)*, it is unlawful to discriminate against workers because of religion or similar belief. This applies to both direct discrimination (that is treating someone less favourably than others because of their religion or belief) and indirect (applying a criterion, provision or practice which disadvantages people of a particular religion or belief without a good reason).

In today's diverse health workforce, disputes in relation to religious practice – for example requests for time off for holy days, or objections to participating in certain health treatments – are widely anticipated. Employers can reduce the risks of disputes and the effect on patient care by:

● Identifying the religions and beliefs which may apply in their workplace

● Raising awareness of different religious observances and their likely impact

● Consulting with their Equalities Group on the incorporation of religion and belief in the equal opportunities, bullying and harassment and other related policies

● Ensuring fair interpretation by training and monitoring

Applying the new regulations in this positive way will add value to an organisation's diversity ethos, and contribute to patient choice and services, by taking account of religion and belief.

Sexual orientation 9.112

Under the new *Employment Equality (Sexual orientation) Regulations 2003 (SI 2003/1661)*, it is unlawful to discriminate against workers because of sexual orientation. This covers direct discrimination (that is, treating someone less favourably because of their actual or perceived sexual orientation), and indirect discrimination (applying a criterion, provision or practice which disadvantages an individual because of their sexual orientation without good reason).

The new regulations also cover harassment and victimisation. Staff who are subject to such discrimination now have a legal remedy, but policies incorporating sexual orientation also make good business sense and reduces risk, as discrimination causes people to be less productive and lose motivation.

Age discrimination 9.113

The EC Equal Treatment Directive (*EC Directive establishing a general framework for equal treatment in employment and occupation 2000/78/EC*) requires the implementation of age discrimination rules by 2006, and the Government has just issued a consultation document[32] with proposals for tackling discrimination and harassment on age grounds.

A central premise of the document is that age discrimination blights employment opportunities for young and old alike. The NHS diversity framework already covers age discrimination, and it is covered in equal opportunity policies. However, the new regulations will enforce these rights in terms of direct and indirect discrimination.

There are increasing claims being made to Employment Tribunals on age grounds, primarily using sex discrimination legislation. Recent cases have covered retirement age, and rights to unfair dismissal or redundancy payments, which currently have an upper age limit. It is important to remain aware of these cases, and apply good employment practices irrespective of age. This will attract staff, add to the profile of the model employer, and reduce the risks.

All employers must have policies to ensure risk reduction from unlawful discrimination acts by managers and staff. All managers must be trained in equality issues, ensure their actions do not infringe legislation and refer any issues arising for specialist human resource advice.

Bullying and harassment 9.114

An increasing area of challenge, which can affect morale and employee attraction and retention, is harassment on grounds of sex or race, sexual orientation or religion and belief. Unless employers have effective policies covering this, and act swiftly to deal with all instances of harassment, whether by patients, managers or staff, they are open to complaints of discrimination. Recent cases show costs can be high, particularly where there is in addition an award for injury to feelings arising out of unlawful discrimination, or a claim for compensation for psychiatric injury or stress.

Human rights 9.115

Employers must also take account of new legislation on civil liberties. The *Human Rights Act 1998* gives the right to challenge public authorities where they act in conflict with human rights. Employment-related rights protected include the right to freedom of expression, association and assembly, and to privacy and family life.

Power to investigate 9.116

The *Regulation of Investigatory Powers Act 2000* limits employers' rights to intercept employee Emails, faxes and telephone calls, unless consent has been given or there is a legitimate business interest. Since increasing reliance is placed on Email as a prime means of business communication, this is a growing area of risk, but the new rules mean employers cannot rely on the right to take action on Email or internet abuse unless policy has been effectively communicated.

Whistle blowing 9.117

Under the *Public Interest Disclosure Act 1998*, an employee who blows the whistle on an employer's fraudulent or criminal activities has protection against victimisation, provided they follow prescribed routes. This will include protection for health workers in situations such as the Bristol case, and be important in the future for enabling unsafe processes to be identified and action taken before they become major issues. All NHS employers must have whistle blowing policies.

A recent report from Public Concern at Work[33] found that people are increasingly likely now to blow the whistle on workplace wrongdoing. The top two issues among callers to the charity's help line are safety risks and financial misconduct. The number of calls from the care sector has recently increased from 5% to 17%.

This emphasises the importance of clinical governance and management systems to avoid poor practice, which may result in public, whistle blowing and affect confidence in local health care.

Excessive working hours 9.118

A key area of risk in clinical practice is long working hours. The *Working Time Regulations 1998 (SI 1998/1833)* came into force on 1 October 1998, implementing the European *Working Time Directive (Council Directive concerning certain aspects of the organisation of working time 93/104/EC)*. It is important to note that the Directive was adopted as a health and safety measure, to ensure minimum rest periods, leave entitlements and maximum weekly working hours protection for all workers.

Working Time Regulations 9.119

Under the Regulations, working time is limited to:

- an average of 48 hours a week over the reference period (generally 26 weeks); and

- an average of eight hours in 24 for night workers.

There are also the following rights:

- for night workers to receive free health assessments;

- to 11 hours' rest in each 24 hours;

- to a rest period of 24 hours in every seven days (or 48 hours in each 14 days);

- to an in-work rest break if the working day is longer than six hours; and

- to four weeks' paid leave per year from day one of employment.

These limits are lower for young workers.

Impact on health organisations   9.120

These rights and obligations have had a considerable impact on the organisation of working time in health organisations, where groups of health workers have a variety of contractual arrangements, including shift and nightwork, on-call and standby, temporary and additional bank work, and overtime. Employers have had to adjust shift patterns and invest in additional employees, to ensure they are able to cover the service and provide the entitled breaks. This is a good example of where the needs of the service will not protect employers from possible prosecution if rest breaks are not provided; the only options may be service reductions, with their own risks, or investment in staff.

Exceptions to the Regulations   9.121

It is the nature of healthcare provision that there will be instances where people will be needed to work beyond the limits – for example, consultants in operating theatres, radiographers called out at night and ambulance paramedics attending an emergency at the end of their shift. The Regulations allow for this in several ways, but there are risks for the employer in ensuring safe working practices.

By virtue of *regulation 4* of the *Working Time Regulations 1998 (SI 1998/1833)*, individual workers can, by written agreement, choose to disapply the weekly working hours limit. In addition, workers whose working time (or part of it) is not measured or predetermined are exempt from some provisions. However, the basis of the Regulations is that long hours are harmful to health. A failure to monitor working time, or to protect against excessive working, could therefore be used as evidence of a failure to provide a safe system of work if an employee brings a claim against their employer. *Johnstone v Bloomsbury Health Authority [1991] 2 All ER 293* illustrates this (see box below).

In the health economy today, many doctors and other professionals still work exceptionally long hours to meet clinical need. Employers must ensure hours and health are monitored to avoid the risk of similar cases.

A case of excessive working hours

Dr Johnstone was a senior house officer employed under a contract of employment with a standard working week of 40 hours and, in addition, availability on call for a further 48 hours a week. He claimed that the authority was under a duty to take all reasonable care for his safety and well-being, and that they were in breach of that duty by requiring him to work intolerable hours. The Court of Appeal ruled that the authority could not lawfully require a doctor to work so much overtime in any week, as it was reasonably foreseeable that it would damage his health.

From August 2004 junior doctors will be required under the *Working Time Directive* provisions to limit their hours of work to no more than 58 per week, including residential on call time. The change management implications of this are explored in **CHAPTER 3**.

Rest periods   9.122

The Regulations also provide for derogation on rest periods in certain specified circumstances or where there is a collective agreement, provided that compensatory rest is given. In the case of career grade doctors, a derogation of some Regulations relating to nightworking and rest has been applied, subject to the provision of compensatory rest

The problem for health employers is ensuring that compensatory rest is given within a reasonable space of time, whilst also protecting clinical activity such as theatre lists. NHS employers have local agreements on this in accordance with national guidance. However, it is clear that there is an expectation from the HSE, and healthcare professionals themselves, that these policies will ensure protection for workers and patients.

There are also problems for employers in preventing excessive hours working by employees with second jobs with another employer. This situation requires careful monitoring to protect patient care. If there is an effect on performance, then action should be taken under fair procedures.

Exit interviews   9.123

An exit interview is a conversation between a departing employee who is leaving either voluntarily or involuntarily, and a representative from the organisation. Although of benefit to employees as a means of identifying complaints, the real value of the exit interview is as a reality check for the employer, to see how the organisation is doing. In terms of risk management, the exit interview is a signifi-cant learning tool, with the opportunity to identify poor or unsafe practice, and to take action before public whistleblowing occurs.

The employee's line manager or supervisor should not conduct the exit inter-view, as they will almost certainly not be sufficiently objective, and may inhibit honest replies. In most cases, properly trained human resources staff are best suited for this role. Questions must be open ended, sensitive, neutral and tailored to each individual in order to identify particular concerns or inconsistencies.

What should the interview cover?   9.124

All exit interviews should be structured to check leaving arrangements, terms and conditions and attitudes to the organisation as an employer. However, an inter-view focusing on risk management must in particular cover:

- reasons for the termination or departure;

- the supervisor's management skills;

- any concerns about working practices;

- how effectively the department operates; and

- any questionable practices connected with the termination or departure – for example, improper payments.

Protecting the organisation   9.125

The exit interview also gives the organisation two further opportunities con-nected with risk management. One is to ensure the employee understands any continuing obligations about confidentiality, and returns any keys, security or identity cards, codes or healthcare property. There may also be a need to resolve any outstanding disputes, and explain policy on the provision of references. There may also be a need to protect the organisation by assessing whether the employee is high risk for any grudge action – for example, computer sabotage – or whether an alert warning to other employers is needed.

Staff retention issues   9.126

The second opportunity is to identify staff retention issues, particularly in areas of recruitment shortages, and how these may be addressed. The exit interview is the last opportunity to persuade people to stay, either in the same role or by rede-ployment in another area, or to return at a later date. Career break schemes, parental leave, elder care, study leave and secondments are all important elements in the make up of a good employer, and will be positive and much cheaper alter-natives to offer to avoid the resignation of a valued employee.

Good practice in people management 9.127

The people issues of risk management in healthcare are constantly evolving, either because of legislative or case law developments, or as a result of changing government or NHS policy. It is essential that health employers keep up to date with these developments, and incorporate them in their policies and the day-to-day management of the organisation. Employers and managers must ensure they have all the relevant documentation, and seek expert human resources or legal advice, before taking action.

Key actions 9.128

So what, in summary are the key actions an employer can take to effectively manage the people risks, and make a real difference to care and business outcomes? The model healthcare employer must have in place a number of key mechanisms (SEE BOX BELOW).

Action along these lines will help ensure that health organisations are more attractive places to work, encouraging recruitment, retention and morale. It will also contribute to the ability to move forward, taking account of lessons from the past, and to greater organisational success for the future.

Key human resource strategies to underpin risk management

- Sound recruitment and selection procedures, including pre-employment checks, training in equality and interview skills and good induction.

- Systems for learning from errors, including blame culture eradication, appraisal and retraining, and for keeping up to date with legislation and other developments.

- Strategies for adequate resourcing, including employee attraction and retention, a balanced skill mix and continuous monitoring of job content and workload through performance review.

- Effective performance based on high-quality teams, high-quality leadership and sound supervision.

- Action to improve morale by good communications and staff involvement.

- A comprehensive range of human resource policies, including those to tackle sickness absence and discrimination.

References

See also KEY REFERENCES, Appendix 1

1 Presentation reported in *HR in the NHS Conference Special*, July 2003
2 DoH (2003), *Delivering the HR in the NHS Plan 2003*, DoH.
3 The Allitt Inquiry (1994) *The Allitt Inquiry, Independent inquiry relating to deaths and injuries on the children's ward at Grantham and Kesteven General Hospital during the period February to April 1991*, HMSO, London.
4 Bullock, R (1997) *Report of the independent inquiry into the major employment and ethical issues arising from the events leading to the trial of Amanda Jenkinson*, North Nottinghamshire Health Authority, Nottingham.
5 Commission for Health Improvement (2001) *Employing locum consultants – matters arising from the employment of Dr Elwood*, CHI, London. (www.chi.nhs.uk)
6 *Code of Practice in HCHS Locum Doctor Appointment and Employment*, NHS Executive, August 1997.
7 HMSO (2002), *Learning from Bristol: the Department of Health's response to the Report of the Public Inquiry into children's heart surgery at the Bristol Royal Infirmary 1984–1995*, (Cm 5363), HMSO.
8 Redfern, M (2001) *The report of The Royal Liverpool Children's Inquiry*, HMSO, London. (www.rlcinquiry.org.uk).
9 The Victoria Climbie Inquiry Report: key findings from the self audits of NHS organisations, social services departments and police forces, Commission for Health Improvement, October 2003
10 Audit Commission (2002), *Recruitment and retention, a public sector workforce for the twenty-first century*, Audit Commission..
11 DoH (2003), *Equalities and diversity strategy and delivery Plan to support the NHS*.
12 Office of the Commissioner for Public Appointments (2001) *OCPA Code of practice for ministerial appointments to public bodies*, OCPA, London. (www.ocpa.gov.uk)
13 Department of Health (2001) *Assuring the quality of medical practice*, HMSO, London.
14 Health Service Circular 2002/003, *Pre and post employment checks for all persons working in the NHS in England*
15 'Sentence served: recruiting ex-offenders', *IRS Employment Review 799*, July 2003.
16 *Breaking the circle, a summary of the views of consultees and the Government response to the report of the review of the Rehabilitation of Offenders Act 1974*, April 2003.
17 The Employment Practices Code Part 4 – information about workers' health, draft for consultation, December 2003.
18 DoH, (2003), *Health Clearance for Serious Communicable Diseases: New Health Care Workers, Draft guidance for consultation*, DoH.
19 Penna Sanders & Sidney (1998), *Surviving the honeymoon: research report*, Penna Sanders & Sidney, London.
20 Department of Health (1999), *Supporting doctors, protecting patients*, HMSO, London.
21 GMC (2003), *New arrangements for GMC Registration and Licensure: A consultation paper*.
22 HSC 2002/011 *The issue of alert letters for health professionals in England*
23 Deeks, E (2001) 'Solitary lessons in how to manage your weaknesses', *People Management*, 17 May.
24 HSE (2001), *Proposals for a new duty to investigate, accidents, dangerous occurrences and diseases*, HSE consultative document (CD 169).
25 DoH (2002), *Code of conduct for NHS Managers*, DoH.
26 Aston Centre for Health Service Organisation Research, *Team Working and Effectiveness in Healthcare – findings from the Health Care Team Effectiveness Project*, Aston University.
27 Department of Health (2001) *Code of practice for NHS employers involved in the international recruitment of healthcare professionals*, DoH, London.

28   Buchan, J (2000) *Determining skill mix in the health workforce: guidelines for managers and health professionals (discussion paper 3)*, World Health Organisation, Geneva.

29   Department of Health (2002) *Recruitment and progression minimising attrition from NHS funded pre-registration healthcare courses*

30   *Employee absence 2003: a survey of management policy and practice*, CIPD, June 2003.

31   Department of Health (2001) *Assuring the quality of medical practice*, HMSO, London.

32   DTI (2003), *Equality and diversity: age matters, age consultation 2003*, DTI.

33   *Two years back, Three years forward, Ten years old*, Public Concern at Work, October 2003.

Appendix I
Key References

The following references are essential background for readers of this handbook. All can be downloaded free of charge from the website addresses given.

Department of Health (1996) *Code of Conduct: Code of Accountability*, HMSO, London

Department of Health (1997) *The New NHS: Modern, Dependable*, HMSO, London (www.doh.gov.uk/nnhsind.htm)

Department of Health (1998) *A First Class Service: Quality in the new NHS*, HMSO, London (www.doh.gov.uk/nnhsind.htm)

Department of Health (2000) *The NHS Plan: A plan for investment, a plan for reform*, HMSO, London (www.doh.gov.uk/nhsplan)

Department of Health (2000) *An Organisation with a Memory*, HMSO, London (www.doh.gov.uk/orgmemreport)

Department of Health (2001) *Building a Safer NHS for Patients*, HMSO, London (www.doh.gov.uk/buildsafenhs)

Department of Health (2001) *Doing Less Harm – Improving the safety and quality of care through reporting, analysing and learning from adverse incidents involving NHS patients* (www.npsa.org.uk)

Department of Health (2001) *Learning from Bristol: the report of the public inquiry into children's heart surgery at the Bristol Royal Infirmary 1984–1995*, Command Paper CM 5207, HMSO, London (www.bristol-inquiry.org.uk)

NHS Executive (1999) *Guidelines for Implementing Controls Assurance in the NHS*, NHSE, Leeds, November 1999 *(www.doh.go.uk/riskman.htm)*. The controls assurance website also features the latest controls assurance standards

Turnbull N and working party (1999) *Internal Control – Guidance for Directors on the Combined Code (The Turnbull Report)*, Institute of Chartered Accountants in England and Wales, London (www.icaew.co.uk/internalcontrol)

271

Appendix 2
Glossary

Adverse healthcare event, an untoward incident associated with healthcare delivery. An event or omission arising during clinical care and causing physical or psychological injury to a patient.

Business continuity management, the process by which arrangements are made to ensure service delivery following major disruption to normal business activity.

Clinical governance, the application of the principles of corporate governance to clinical risk, with the overall aim of enhancing the quality of patient care delivery.

Clinical risk, risk specifically associated with clinical practice or patient care delivery.

Clinical risk management, a systematic process where clinical risk is identified and measures introduced to reduce risk with the overall aim of improving patient care.

Continuous professional development, the development of personal pro-grammes of training and development for professional staff, including clinicians and healthcare staff, to ensure their professional practice remains up to date.

Controls assurance, the approach to corporate governance developed within the NHS. A verification process to test that NHS organisations are effectively managing risk.

Corporate governance, a holistic approach to developing systems of internal control within an organisation and to the verification of the effectiveness of these systems.

Credentialling, the verification during recruitment of an individual's identity, qualifications and experience in order to ensure the quality of healthcare provision.

Crisis management, the strategic response in the immediate aftermath of a major incident.

Drug error, a mistake in administration of patient medication.

Error, a mistake either intended or unintended that leads to an adverse outcome. Errors can be both active and have immediate effect or latent where the consequences become apparent after a period of time.

Hazard, the potential to cause harm.

Hazard identification, the process by which hazards are determined or spotted.

Human factors, environmental, organisational and job factors, and human and individual characteristics which influence behaviour at work in a way that can affect risk.

Incident, undesired circumstances which may or may not cause harm.

Near-miss, an accident with the potential to cause harm or damage.

Risk, the probability or chance that harm will arise.

Risk assessment, the systematic identification of the causes of harm and additional measures necessary to remove or reduce risk.

Risk management, the systematic identification, evaluation and treatment of risk. A continuous process with the aim of reducing risk to organisations and individuals alike.

Root cause, the immediate underlying cause of an incident or accident that can be readily identified and is within the ability of managers and staff to fix.

Service continuity management, a term interchangeable with business continuity management, most usually used in service organisations.

Service continuity plans, the identification of the systematic steps to be planned and followed in order to ensure continuity of service provision.

Service recovery, a term interchangeable with business recovery, involving the arrangements to be put in place to ensure continuity of service provision following major disruption.

Skill mix, the blend of skills needed amongst a team of staff to ensure effective healthcare delivery.

Supply chain, the interdependent relationship between organisations supplying goods and services.

Table of Cases

Table of Statutes

Table of Statutory Instruments

Table of European Legislation

Index

Index

Index

National Patient Safety Agency (NPSA) – *contd*

An Organisation with a Memory (OWAM) 4.54, 5.23, 6.71, 9.71

Seven steps to patient safety 4.4, 5.24, 5.25

National Programme for IT 4.52

National Reporting and Learning System (NRLS) 5.23, 5.24

national service frameworks (NSFs) 2.6, 2.33

National Shared Services Initiative 3.36

New NHS: Modern, Dependable, The 2.26

NHS Direct 9.84

NHS Estates 3.36, 7.4, 7.68

NHS Plan 9.4
- alternative staffing solutions 9.83
- buildings 7.4, 7.34
- organisational change 3.4
- regulatory bodies, reform of 3.9
- workforce expansion 9.5, 9.79

NHS Professionals 9.54, 9.80

NHS Supplies 3.36

NHS University 3.8

night work
- *Hospital at Night* 3.42

non-clinical risk 2.14, 6.71

non-clinical staff
- generally 9.100
- Health Professionals Council 9.101
- new roles and policies 9.105
- operating department practitioners 9.102
- recruitment and selection 9.103
- under-investment, impact of 9.104

Nursing and Midwifery and Allied Health Professionals Council 3.9

O

occupational health 6.69–6.70
- *see also* pre-employment occupational health screening

Ombudsman *see* Health Service Ombudsman

operating department practitioners (ODPs) 9.102

Organisation with a Memory, An (OWAM) 4.54, 5.23, 6.71, 8.10, 9.71

organisational change
- Care Trusts 3.39
- drivers for change 3.4–3.5
- employee relations, and 3.15
- Foundation Trusts 3.38

organisational change – *contd*
- General Medical Services (GMS) contract 3.40
- generally 3.1
- junior doctors' hours 3.42
- learning organisations 3.2
- legal framework 3.17–3.27
- liabilities, transfer of 3.29
- mergers of Trusts 3.29, 3.34
- models of 3.2–3.3
- morale, and 3.12
- new consultant contract 3.41
- NHS Plan 3.5
- organisational health, and 3.12
- outsourcing 3.18, 3.36
- pace of 3.13
- pay and conditions, role of 3.14
- people management
  - generally 3.6
  - learning and personal development 3.8
  - pay and rewards 3.7
  - regulation 3.9
  - workforce planning 3.10
- Primary Care Groups (PCGs) 3.35
- Primary Care Trusts (PCTs) 3.35, 3.39, 3.40
- Private Finance Initiative (PFI) 3.28
  - transfer of liabilities 3.29
- project management 3.3
- psychological contract, and 3.16
- risks of
  - employee relations 3.15
  - generally 3.11
  - morale 3.12
  - organisational health 3.12
  - pace of change 3.13
  - pay and conditions, role of 3.14
  - psychological contract 3.16
- shared services 3.36
- Shifting the Balance of Power (STBOP) 3.37
- SWOT analysis 3.2
- transfer of liabilities 3.29
- transfer of undertakings
  - collective agreements 3.23
  - consultation 3.25
  - contracts of employment 3.18, 3.24
  - dismissals 3.18
  - identifying existence of 3.18
  - pensions 3.20, 3.27
- Public Private Partnerships (PPPs) 3.26, 3.27
- public sector transfers 3.26
- redundancy 3.18, 3.21

290